M. *Sandra Wood, MLS, MBA*
Editor

Health Care Resources
on the Internet
A Guide for Librarians
and Health Care Consumers

Pre-publication
REVIEW

"**A** practical field guide and an essential research tool to the Internet's vast and varied resources for health care has arrived—and its voice is professional and accessible. Sandy Wood has assembled a dream team of seventeen health science reference librarian experts to share their collective Net savvy and research wisdom. This 'everything you need to know' comprehensive work is an important reference tool that is readable and enjoyable. Scholars will appreciate the thorough documentation, a model for citing all things cyber. Practicing librarians will bookmark the cite recommendations for sure. Students and teachers of health information will welcome this book as a text that is clear and current. Consumers will benefit from something not often found among other 'hype'-type guides—a considered and evaluative approach.

The core overview essays on reference today, on searching the Net, and on MEDLINE are well written and important background. The topical chapters on alternative medicine, government resources, statistical information, and international health are rich with recommendations and advice derived from practice. These topics are the 'hot' lunchtime/cocktail party concerns of all involved with health care today. This little book is 'cool'! It's reasoned, seasoned, and validation that for their health care Internet 'smarts,' librarians rule as consumer information advisors. Responsible patients and eager consumers will learn well to navigate and will thank Ms. Wood."

Elizabeth R. Warner, MSLS, AHIP
Coordinator of Information Literacy Programs, Academic Information Services and Research, Thomas Jefferson University, Philadelphia, PA

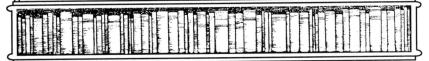

Health Care Resources on the Internet

A Guide for Librarians and Health Care Consumers

Health Care Resources on the Internet
A Guide for Librarians and Health Care Consumers

M. Sandra Wood, MLS, MBA
Editor

The Haworth Information Press
New York • London • Oxford

Published by

The Haworth Information Press, an imprint of The Haworth Press, Inc., 10 Alice Street, Binghamton, NY 13904-1580

Cover design by Marylouise E. Doyle.

Library of Congress Cataloging-in-Publication Data

Health care resources on the internet : a guide for librarians and health care consumers / M. Sandra Wood, editor.
  p. cm.
 Includes bibliographical references and index.
 ISBN 0-7890-0632-4 (alk. paper). — ISBN 0-7890-0911-0 (pbk. : alk. paper).
 1. Medicine—Computer network resources. 2. Internet (Computer network). 3. Medical care—Computer network resources. 4. Medical informatics. I. Wood, M. Sandra. II. Title: Guide for librarians and health care consumers.
R119.9.H39 1999
025.06′61—dc21
                               99-37569
                                   CIP

CONTENTS

ABOUT THE EDITOR

M. Sandra Wood, MLS, MBA, is Librarian, Reference and Database Services at The Milton S. Hershey Medical Center at The Pennsylvania State University of Hershey, Pennsylvania. She holds the academic rank of librarian and has over twenty-nine years of experience as a medical reference librarian, including the areas of general reference services, management of reference services, database and Internet searching, and user instruction. Ms. Wood has been widely published in the field of medical reference and is Editor of the journal *Medical Reference Services Quarterly* (Haworth) and Editor of *Health Care on the Internet* (Haworth). She is a member of the Medical Library Association and the Special Libraries Association, and has served on MLA's Board of Directors as Treasurer. Ms. Wood is also a Fellow of the Medical Library Association.

Contributors

Nancy J. Allee, BA, MLS, MPH, is Director of Public Health Information Services and Access (PHISA) at the University of Michigan, Ann Arbor, Michigan, a position she has held since April 1997. PHISA is responsible for providing network, computing, library, and Web services for the School of Public Health. She is chair of the Public Health Training Subcommittee of the Joint Centers for Disease Control/National Library of Medicine Public Health Initiative, a past president of the Public Health/Health Administration Section of the Medical Library Association, a member of the Academy of Health Information Professionals, and a recipient of the ACE (Agent for Cooperative Efforts) Award from the University of Michigan Library.

helen-ann brown, MLS, MS, teaches MEDLINE as a member of the Information Services Team of the Cornell Medical Library of the Weill Medical College in New York City. Her career as a health sciences librarian spans more than twenty-five years. Her professional career began in Washington, DC, at the Walter Reed Army Medical Center. She was the first full-time clinical librarian at the Tompkins McCaw Library of the Medical College of Virginia, Richmond, Virginia. At the National Jewish Center in Denver, she directed the Library and continued her clinical librarianship for adult medicine as well as pediatrics. helen-ann has taught thousands of people to search MEDLINE as Online Coordinator of the Midlands Online Region of the National Network of Libraries of Medicine, and as a BRS trainer.

Nancy Calabretta, MEd, MS, is a health sciences librarian with over twenty-six years of experience. She is currently Reference Librarian at the Reuben L. Sharp Health Science Library, the Cooper Health System, Camden, New Jersey. She has been an adjunct professor at Drexel's College of Information Science and Technology, Philadelphia, Pennsylvania, since 1985.

Janet M. Coggan, BS, MEd, MSLS, worked as the Area Health Education Center Coordinator in the Reference Department of the University of Florida Health Science Center (HSC) Library, Gainesville, Florida, for nine years, until Fall 1998. During that time, Coggan was very active in the Consumer and Patient Health Information Section of the Medical Library Association and developed a consumer health collection for the HSC Library. In addition, she served as the editor of the book review column for *Medical Reference Services Quarterly* for three years and currently serves as the book review editor for the *Bulletin of the Medical Library Association.* She has published numerous book reviews and articles in professional journals and newsletters.

Esther Y. Dell, BA, AMLS, is Assistant Librarian, the George T. Harrell Library, Milton S. Hershey Medical Center, Pennsylvania State University, Hershey, Pennsylvania. She has a longtime interest in alternative medical therapy and has followed the development of this practice, both in print and on the Internet, as the literature expands and evolves. Over the last several years, she has worked with Suzanne M. Shultz and Nancy I. Henry in making presentations, and delivering speeches, and writing papers on alternative medicine. She and Nancy I. Henry edit a column titled "Alternative and Complementary Therapy" in the journal *Health Care on the Internet.*

Eric P. Delozier, BS, MLS, is Assistant Librarian for Reference and Electronic Services, Heindel Library, Penn State Harrisburg, Middletown, Pennsylvania. Delozier is editor of the journal, *Health Care on the Internet,* has served as column editor of "Navigate the Net" for *Medical Reference Services Quarterly,* and is the author of numerous articles about searching the Internet.

Cindy A. Gruwell, BA, MLS, is Assistant Librarian/Coordinator of Outreach, Twin Cities Bio-Medical Library, University of Minnesota, Minneapolis, Minnesota. Following a career change from retail management to librarianship in 1995, Gruwell joined the University Libraries at the University of Minnesota, Twin Cities, as a post-MLS resident. In January 1996, she assumed the position of Assistant Librarian and Outreach Coordinator for the Bio-Medical Library, with duties that include reference, bibliographic instruction, and outreach/public relations to health science students, staff, and faculty of the university.

Nancy I. Henry, MLS, is Assistant Librarian, Life Sciences Library, Pattee Library, Pennsylvania State University, University Park, Pennsylvania. She has a longtime interest in alternative medical therapy and has followed the development of this practice, both in print and on the Internet, as the literature expands and evolves. Over the last several years, she has worked with Suzanne M. Shultz and Esther Y. Dell in making presentations, and delivering speeches, and writing papers on alternative medicine. She and Esther Y. Dell edit a column titled "Alternative and Complementary Therapy" in the journal *Health Care on the Internet.*

Virginia A. Lingle, BS, MSLS, is Associate Librarian, Cataloging, Serials, and Collection Development, the George T. Harrell Library, Milton S. Hershey Medical Center, Pennsylvania State University, Hershey, Pennsylvania. Lingle has worked with implementing electronic access to journals for end users for the last several years and has organized programs for the Collection Development Section of the Medical Library Association on the topic.

Dawn M. Littleton, MLS, MA, is a reference librarian at the University of Minnesota, Twin Cities Bio-Medical Library, Minneapolis, Minnesota, where she has been the education technology coordinator and an instructor of World Wide Web searching strategies and resources in statistics.

Scott Marsalis, MLS, BA, is Information Services Librarian, Biomedical Information Service, Twin Cities Bio-Medical Library, University of Minnesota, Minneapolis, Minnesota. He has held positions as a cataloger and reference librarian at the Minnesota Historical Society and was Corporate Librarian for ReliaStar Financial for three years. In 1998, Mr. Marsalis joined the University of Minnesota's Bio-Medical Library as an Information Services

Librarian. He splits his duties between the BioMedical Information Service, primarily doing online searches for nonuniversity clients, and the reference department.

Alexa Mayo, MSLS, is an information specialist and the Coordinator of Education and Publications at the University of Maryland, Health Sciences and Human Services Library, Baltimore, Maryland. She previously has worked in a hospital library and as an academic reference librarian at the College of the Holy Cross in Worcester, Massachusetts.

Cynthia R. Phyillaier, MSLS, is an information specialist at the Health Sciences and Human Services Library, University of Maryland, Baltimore. Prior to becoming an information specialist, she worked for many years as a registered respiratory therapist in critical care.

Valerie G. Rankow, BA, MLS, has been a professional librarian for nearly thirty years, in a career that includes public service and administrative positions in academic health science, special and public libraries, as well as a private information consulting business. She presently brings that experience into cyberspace as the Medical Cybrarian for HealthWorld Online (http://www.healthy.net/library/cybrarian/index.html). Valerie worked as an award-winning professional writer, specializing in health and medicine, and is an adjunct faculty member at a local professional library, where she teaches continuing education classes and training workshops.

Jeri Ann Risin, MLIS, is a researcher at LAI Worldwide and is a member of the Special Libraries Association and Suncoast Information Specialists. Risin was an information specialist for two years in the Medical Devices Research Division at HSBC Securities in Clearwater, Florida.

Kathryn Robbins, MLIS, PhD, is a reference librarian at the University of Minnesota, Twin Cities Bio-Medical Library, Minneapolis, Minnesota, where she has been Head of Reference Desk Services for the past eight years.

Suzanne M. Shultz is Director of Library Services, the Philip A Hoover, MD, Library, York Health System, York, Pennsylvania.

She has a longtime interest in alternative medical therapy and has followed the development of this practice, both in print and on the Internet, as the literature expands and evolves. Over the last several years, she has worked with Nancy I. Henry and Esther Y. Dell in making presentations, and delivering speeches, and writing papers on alternative medicine.

Introduction

M. Sandra Wood

The way in which we find information has been transformed over the past five years by the Internet. Both end users and librarians have come to rely on the World Wide Web (WWW) for answers to factual questions and as a resource for current information. One can find everything from the weather, stock market quotes, or late-breaking news to online textbooks, encyclopedias, and databases. Whereas users previously had come to the library to research a topic using print sources such as textbooks and indexes, they now can search online from the comfort of their own homes or offices, or they will come to the library to "surf the Net." Reference librarians are constantly being asked, "Can't you find it on the Internet?"—even before the patron actually indicates what subject he or she is seeking. Frequently, the user has already done a preliminary search on the Internet and, if unable to locate what he or she wants, will ask the reference librarian either to take the search further or to verify that nothing else can be found.

In the medical and health care arena, access to medical information has become highly dependent on the Internet. All users of medical information, from researchers and clinicians to health care consumers, are using the Internet to locate answers to their questions. As more users raise their expectations of what they can find on the Internet, they have looked to health sciences librarians to be experts in searching the WWW. Rather than going to the shelf to find a directory or textbook to answer a question, librarians are accessing the WWW to locate the appropriate information for their users or they are reciting URLs (uniform resource locators) from memory to guide their patrons to appropriate locations to find the information for themselves. The "core collection" traditionally maintained at the reference/information desk is being supplemented and/or replaced by appropriate Web sites that have

been bookmarked for ready, online access. Such sites include professional associations (e.g., the American Medical Association at http://
www.ama-assn.org), bibliographic databases (e.g., MEDLINE via
PubMed at http://www.nlm.nih.gov), consumer health sites (e.g.,
NOAH: New York Online Access to Health at http://www.noah.
cuny.edu), medical textbooks (e.g., Harrison's Online at http://www.
harrisonsonline.com), and full-text journals (e.g., *APA Monitor Online*
at http://www.apa.org/monitor/).

Information on the Internet is constantly changing and being
updated. Web pages are revised, and Web addresses change. Immediate access to current information is the greatest strength of the
Internet; however, this strength is at the same time its major weak-
ness. Despite search engines to help users locate information, the
Internet has grown, unregulated, at such a fast pace that there is no
simple, ordered way to approach a search. Material of questionable
content is retrieved right along with high-quality information; a
Web site comes up one day, only to be missing the next (who hasn't
gotten the message "URL not found at this location"?). Smart users
need to assess the information that they find on the WWW, looking,
for example, at the source (who provided it and what expertise do
they have?) and at how current it is (when was the Web page last
updated?). All Web sites are *not* "created equal," and users of the
Internet are urged to evaluate information critically before using it.
Health care consumers should consult their physicians when in
doubt about the appropriateness of treatment information found on
the Internet.

*Health Care Resources on the Internet: A Guide for Librarians and
Health Care Consumers* is intended as an introduction to finding
health care information on the Internet. Rather than simply providing
an annotated list of recommended Web sites, this volume emphasizes
how to search efficiently for quality information. Throughout the volume, readers are guided to recommended sites and given tips on where
to begin their search through the maze of information found on the
Web.

In Chapter 1, "Use of the Internet at the Reference Desk," Nancy
Calabretta describes the current state of reference, emphasizing the
use of Internet resources and the World Wide Web at the reference
desk. The Internet has become an invaluable tool for finding health

care information, and librarians will rely more and more on this source of information into the twenty-first century.

In Chapter 2, "Natural Language and Beyond: Tips for Search Services," Eric P. Delozier gives practical tips on how to use Internet search services effectively. He divides search services into three categories: engines (e.g., HotBot, Excite, AltaVista), subject directories (e.g., Yahoo!, Galaxy), and metasearch gateways (e.g., MetaCrawler, Dogpile). Search tips include using more than one search service.

Cindy A. Gruwell and Scott Marsalis overview "Megasites for Health Care Information" in Chapter 3. Their advice includes evaluating the quality of the site and using the sites as starting points or links to other sites. An annotated list of megasites is divided by sites for consumers, sites that are "information intensive," with few links, and sites for medical professionals.

Journals form the "heart" of the biomedical literature. For this reason, an entire chapter is devoted to MEDLINE, the premier database of the National Library of Medicine. In Chapter 4, "MEDLINE on the Internet," helen-ann brown and Valerie G. Rankow discuss the basics of how to search MEDLINE, including conceptualizing your search, Boolean search formulation, use of MeSH subject headings and textwords, and actual input of the search topic. They overview selected Web-based MEDLINE systems available on the Internet. A section for searching evidence-based medicine is provided for advanced searchers.

In Chapter 5, "Searching the Internet for Diseases," Alexa Mayo and Cynthia R. Phyillaier provide the general framework for searching for virtually any disease on the Internet. Realizing that it is impossible to list all Web sites for all diseases, they have selected examples to illustrate the strategy of searching on the Web. After discussing the kinds and quality of information available, they illustrate how to search for a common disease (lung cancer is used as the example), less common diseases (e.g., Lyme disease), and rare and emerging diseases (e.g., Binswanger's disease). Since consumers might be looking for new treatments, they include a section on searching for open clinical trials.

Janet M. Coggan overviews "Consumer Health Information on the Internet" in Chapter 6. This chapter is intended specifically for patients or health care consumers. Strategies for searching the Net are provided, along with information on how to evaluate a Web site for quality of information. The chapter concludes with some recommended sites where consumers can begin their search.

Recognizing that health care consumers and librarians might not be looking for conventional medical treatments, Suzanne M. Shultz, Nancy I. Henry, and Esther Y. Dell overview accessing information outside the scope of mainstream medicine. In Chapter 7, "Alternative Medicine on the Net," they describe the kinds of electronic resources (e.g., scholarly, pamphlets, promotional, etc.) and give suggestions of good sites to access. Criteria are presented for evaluating the quality of a Web site.

A major source of information on the Internet is the government. In Chapter 8, "Government Resources on the Net," Nancy Allee discusses locating Web-based information from international, federal, and state governments. Emphasis is on U.S. government information, however. The annotated bibliography, based heavily on government agency sites, describes contents of the various Web sites.

Chapter 9, "Health-Related Statistical Information on the Net," by Dawn M. Littleton and Kathryn Robbins, first discusses general strategies for finding health care statistics on the Internet. The chapter is primarily an annotated list of recommended Web sites in two sections: geographical region, listed by international, national, state, and metropolitan, and special topics, listed by disease/subject. Many of these sites are government agencies or professional organizations. Metasites, databases, and search engines are also addressed as sources of statistical information.

In Chapter 10, "Electronic Journals on the Internet," Virginia A. Lingle describes the challenge of finding full-text journal information in magazines and journals on the Internet. More and more, users are expecting to find full-text information on the Net, and they need to be aware that not all information is free. Some sites provide full text, some just abstracts or tables of contents service. Often, there are many access routes to the same journal, and users must navigate through registration requirements, fees, and so forth, to find what they want.

In Chapter 11, "Searching International Medical Resources on the World Wide Web," Jeri Ann Risin introduces Web sites from a variety of locations around the world. Sites for this annotated bibliography were selected to illustrate quality information on the international level.

A caution to all readers of this volume is that, due to constant changes on the Internet, it is inevitable that the URL for many Web sites listed in this book will have changed by the time of publication. This is to be expected. However, using the search principles/ strategies described in this volume should help you to locate the new Web address.

In each chapter, emphasis is placed on evaluating the information that you locate on the Internet. Before you use information found on the Internet, be sure of the source—Where does it come from? Is the source authoritative? How current is it? The smart Internet searcher will be a discriminating Internet consumer.

Although it was not possible (or practical) to try to list every good site that might be used to find health care information, I am hopeful that the search strategies outlined in this volume will help users of the WWW, including librarians, health professionals, and health care consumers, to locate quality information relevant to their needs.

Chapter 1

Use of the Internet at the Reference Desk

Nancy Calabretta

What is it like to be a reference librarian in the late twentieth century? How has the electronic revolution changed the way we do our work as well as the clientele we serve? Two traditional criteria for reference excellence are efficiency and effectiveness. In other words, can you locate good information quickly with little wasted effort? These criteria have been sorely tested by the arrival of the Internet and its resources at the reference desk. The print tools librarians have relied upon for years still exist, of course, but they have been augmented by the arrival of a seemingly unlimited range of electronic resources available through the Internet and its Web. Book and journal budgets now are shared with networked CD-ROM tools and Web subscriptions, while index tables make way for more carrels housing hardware that is perpetually in need of an upgrade. Tenopir and Ennis, continuing research on print versus electronic reference tools begun in the early 1990s, note that "throughout the 1990s, reference departments . . . have seen a rapid evolution from a print-centered world to a digital-intensive one . . . reference librarians expect constant change and have become adept at juggling a vast array of print and online resources."[1] Although this research has focused on academic libraries, it is easy to see parallel trends in public as well as special libraries.

"It was the best of times, it was the worst of times. . . ."[2] The opening lines of Dickens' *A Tale of Two Cities*, set on the eve of the French Revolution, describe very well the positive and negative implications of Web searching, in particular, for reference work. One

1

of the earliest challenges in this evolving electronic environment was for reference librarians themselves to quickly become proficient in using this new and apparently out-of-control tool. The professional literature, meetings, conferences, and continuing education sessions all weighed in heavily on the topic, as those who mastered various aspects of the electronic world shared their skills. Listservs such as MEDLIB-L[3] allowed instant communication of questions and problems, as well as new insights, to colleagues around the world. Now, many useful online guides and tutorials, often created by librarians, exist to guide new users through their beginning attempts at searching. Two excellent examples of such resources are "Finding Information on the Internet: A Tutorial"[4] from the Library at University of California, Berkeley, and "Nothing but 'Net: An Internet Search Guide for Health Professionals" from the J. Otto Lottes Health Science Library, University of Missouri.[5]

Librarians have further responded to this new medium by applying their well-honed information-seeking skills to create compilations of evaluated sites, some of which can be found at HealthWeb,[6] the Librarians' Index to the Internet,[7] and the Internet Public Library.[8] Ironically, these guides are available for easy and immediate sharing due to the electronic medium that they seek to tame. The Internet has made simple a combined effort that was previously possible only through collegial exchanges between institutions or through the more formalized efforts supported by professional groups such as the Public Services Section of the Medical Library Association (MLA).

An experienced Web searcher and librarian who writes frequently about the Internet in reference, Janet Balas reiterates that "reference librarians *must* [emphasis mine] learn how to use the various search engines to their best advantage. This is a daunting task since, like the Internet itself, these search engines are constantly changing."[9] Change is not the only factor to consider. A study of six popular search engines by computer scientists at the NEC Research Institute in Princeton, New Jersey, demonstrated that

the coverage of any one engine is significantly limited: No single search engine indexes more than about one-third of the "indexable Web," the coverage of the six engines investigated varies by an order of magnitude, and combining the results of the six engines yields about 3.5 times as many documents on average as compared with the results from only one engine.[10] [Note: the search engines investigated were HotBot,[11] AltaVista,[12] Excite,[13] Infoseek,[14] Lycos,[15] and Northern Light.[16]]

The current recommendation is to know well and use frequently at least two search engines, with a constant eye toward evaluating both their effectiveness in locating information and any changes in features. It is also necessary to monitor new entries into the field, especially those with a unique approach. For example, Northern Light searches both the Web and its own, full-text "special collection" of articles available by subscription at a very reasonable rate, while Ask Jeeves[17] attempts to answer questions, providing a one-site response, rather than providing a list of sites that meet a specified set of search criteria. Librarians at the University of California, Berkeley, recommend beginning each search by using a metasearch engine, such as MetaFind,[18] Inference Find,[19] Dogpile,[20] or Meta-Crawler,[21] that can query five or more popular search engines at one time. More specific searches can then be done on each search engine that proves to be a good resource for the topic at hand. Metasearch engines can also be used as a last resort tactic in cases when the favorite search engines just don't deliver. The Search Engine Watch site[22] is a good aid for learning about search engines and should be monitored regularly for current awareness. Search Engine Showdown,[23] a site maintained by Greg Notess, is also worth a visit. Notess is "On the Net" columnist for both *ONLINE* and *DATABASE*, as well as reference librarian at Montana State University.

Evaluation is an integral part of using the Internet to provide reference service. Obviously, there is a great deal of concern for the currency, accuracy, and authoritativeness of health care information in particular. The editors of *JAMA* note that

> The Net—and especially the Web—has the potential to become the world's largest vanity press. It is a medium in which anyone with a computer can serve simultaneously as author, editor, and publisher and can fill any or all of these roles anonymously if he or she so chooses.[24]

Many groups have come forward on the issue of quality. The Health On the Net (HON) Foundation,[25] based in Switzerland, has produced and revised the HONCode of Conduct for Medical and Health Web Sites.[26] The HONCode has an accompanying symbol that can be displayed on sites that choose to voluntarily comply with the code. The Health Information Technology Institute of Mitretek Systems, Incorporated, provided the impetus for "White Paper: Criteria for Assessing the Quality of Health Information on the Internet,"[27] a collaborative effort at producing a reliable set of criteria that consumers can use to assess the quality of Internet health information. A group including medical publishers, pharmaceutical companies, patient advocates, medical Internet developers, as well as others, the Internet Healthcare Coalition[28] sponsored the conference "Quality Healthcare Information on the 'Net '98: Delivering on the Promise,"[29] October 5 and 6, 1998, which brought together many of the key players in this arena.

As early participants in efforts to evaluate electronic information resources, librarians logically employed many of the same techniques that had traditionally been used to evaluate print tools. James Rettig, whose popular "Rettig on Reference" reviews[30] are now available on the Web, offered a comparative view of evaluation criteria for print versus electronic resources in "Beyond Cool: Analog Models for Reviewing Digital Resources." [31] A recent effort by Anderson and colleagues,[32] presented at the Medical Library Association Annual Meeting in May 1998, evaluated twenty-five health information megasites. Included among the valuable material at this site is "Checklist of Criteria Used for Evaluation of Megasites," which elucidates key points to consider in three areas—design, content, administrative and quality control. A comprehensive "webliography" titled "Print and Internet Sources on Web Design and Internet Resources Evaluation" can also be found at this site.

Even after experiencing the stress of a rapidly changing dynamic at the reference desk caused by the necessity of learning both new skills and new ways to think about information, the question many reference librarians are asking is "How did we do reference before the Web?"[33] This quote is from Irene McDermott, a reference librarian and frequent contributor to *Searcher*, but the same question has been posed often by colleagues at the Cooper Health System, as we marvel over our latest and greatest triumphs: a list of all consumer products containing latex for the mother of a latex-sensitive toddler; the International Consortium on Jellyfish Stings for a physician treating the aftereffects of a Portuguese Man-of-War sting; the full text of a *Good Housekeeping* article written by a dietitian rating popular diets for a hospital dietitian; reams of material on the medical implications of tattooing and body piercing for the school nurse at a local high school; an exact quote from Dickens' *A Christmas Carol* for the hospital's CEO; the full text of the *Young Parkinson's Handbook* for family members of a thirty-five-year-old woman stricken with Parkinson's disease. Surely, most reference librarians who are actively using the Internet for reference could compile similar lists! McDermott remarks further on our newest, biggest resource, saying, "Even if our library had all the money in the world, we would never have enough space to store all the print resources to cover what the Web gives us at the click of a mouse."[33] The hospital library at the Cooper Health System (and any library with an Internet connection) now has access to a reference collection to rival that of a major university through sites such as the Electronic Reference Shelf from the University of Southern California[34] or the Virtual Reference Desk from Purdue University Libraries.[35] Reference staff can surf over to the Ready Reference Collection of the Internet Public Library[36] rather than calling the public library for answers to general reference queries that were once considered outside the scope of our collection and, sometimes, our expertise. Now, when stumped by a request, the librarians can turn to a worldwide and worldly wise group of colleagues through listservs such as MEDLIB-L. Similarly, librarians working alone in small libraries now have an infinite array of "electronic colleagues" with whom they can discuss problems, seek solutions, and share experiences.

The clientele that is served at the reference desk has also begun to change. There has been a well-documented rise in health consumerism supported by advocates in positions of power. Vice President Gore, in a March 1995 memorandum to Department of Health and Human Services (DHHS) Secretary Donna Shalala, requested that DHHS develop recommendations for providing enhanced consumer health information through the national health information infrastructure. One outcome of this request was *healthfinder*,[37] a gateway site to resources from government and nonprofit organizations, released by DHHS in April 1997 and rereleased in an enhanced version one year later. Gore's announcement of free, Web-based access to MEDLINE in the form of PubMed[38] followed on June 26, 1998. The Vice President noted, at that press conference, "Already, 30,000 people a day are using MEDLINE. By making it more accessible—free and private—we can increase that number many times over."[39] In fact, it took only a few months for this predication to come true. According to the National Library of Medicine (NLM),

> Web usage now accounts for more than 90 percent of all MEDLINE searches done at NLM. The number of searches done on PubMed and Internet Grateful Med in March 1998 was 7.6 million, more than the number of MEDLINE searches done for the whole of 1996 (7.4 million).[40]

In addition, a full 30 percent of those searches are being done by the general public, a development fully supported by renowned heart surgeon Michael E. DeBakey. DeBakey, who is Chair of the NLM Board of Regents, stated,

> Medical breakthroughs are happening so rapidly that I believe health care professionals and consumers alike should be able to tap into the most recent medical information. Even with our modern advances in health care, I still consider good information to be the best medicine.[40]

There has been a growing tendency, therefore, in both hospital and academic libraries, to view the consumer as a really legitimate client, to realize that many consumers can and do move beyond the general and superficial level of information to become "lay experts" in their areas of interest. This development demands a whole different approach to health consumers as users of our reference services. They can no longer be directed to the patient education collection to browse for whatever book or pamphlet may discuss their subjects. Instead, consumers must be guided through their searches for experts in treating rare disorders, complications, or injuries; for the latest treatment breakthroughs; for material to help them evaluate the care they are receiving; for what to expect in the days to come after serious injury or diagnosis; for help in finding rehabilitation facilities, support groups, or even financial advice in dealing with medical crisis situations. As well-known consumer health information expert Alan M. Rees notes,

> The information needs of consumers have become more complex resulting from the momentous changes in the health care delivery system. . . . Choice is highly valued in the selections of options. . . . Choice is, however, relatively meaningless without accurate and reliable information.[41]

Programs sponsored by the Consumer and Patient Health Information Section (CAPHIS) and the Research Section at MLA '98 featured presentations that attempted to answer the question "Consumer Health Information Services: Do They Make a Difference?"[42-44] Services described varied in scope, delivery, and target audiences as well as in the types of libraries offering the services. Additionally, on July 28, 1998, the National Library of Medicine announced a pilot project, Medical Questions? MEDLINE Has Answers, with public libraries "designed to increase public awareness of and access to health information via the Internet."[45] The Medical Library Association, the Public Library Association, the National Network of Libraries of Medicine, the Friends of NLM and the W.K. Kellogg Foundation are partners with NLM on the Medical Questions campaign. MEDLINE*plus*, a consumer health Web site offering access to PubMed as well as information on a growing list of diseases and conditions, was launched by NLM in support of this project on October 22, 1998.[46]

Many health sciences libraries have seen their client bases expand over the past decade. The Internet is a major resource in helping to meet the needs of this user group. As Rees states,

> Libraries that offer the most comprehensive access will be rated at least as highly as those that have the most in-house publications. What is required is not mammoth CHI [consumer health information] collections but rather library staff skilled in knowing where and how to obtain relevant material. This will mean an enhanced role for the librarian to serve as guide, consultant,

advisor, navigator, educator, and Web designer in addition to that of collection specialist. The objective of the library professional will increasingly be to assist part-time (amateur) information searchers in seeking information.[41]

What are some further implications of using the Internet at the reference desk? Librarians can also use the Internet to receive queries as well as to find answers and information. Fishman[47] reviews the literature on using electronic mail at the reference desk, emphasizing the management considerations. The obvious advantages—ease of access at any hour and the potential to build a database of frequently asked questions (FAQs)—are considered in contrast to challenges such as the length of time it takes to answer a question or even complete the reference interview, the lack of nonverbal cues, and the difficulty in sharing the responsibilities among reference staff.

A further enhancement of electronic reference service could include the ability to provide users with search strategy advice at the point of need. OVID's Ask a Librarian feature is one example of such a service, whereby searchers of OVID databases can ask for help with searching problems directly through the OVID search screen. An interesting variation on this type of service is provided at the Norris Medical Library at the University of Southern California, Los Angeles, where students can forward their search strategies online to librarians for assistance.[48]

An extreme example of an electronic reference service is found at the Internet Public Library (IPL), described as an "entirely virtual operation." Lagace and McClennen note that the original IPL reference group, while planning the service,

> kept as our anchor the well-understood process of running a traditional reference desk: providing a visible contact point at which patrons can obtain help in navigating the library's spaces, finding answers to their questions, and evaluating resources. Our conclusion was (and is) that these services are as useful in a virtual environment as in a physical one. . . . [49]

At IPL, staff members, volunteer librarians, and library students answer questions submitted via either the IPL Web form[50] or by e-mail. Questions are routed to a locally developed software system called QRC, which is perhaps one of the most interesting aspects of the project for librarians. QRC (called Quirk by IPL staff) allows for sorting and categorizing the questions as they arrive through its "Incoming Questions" category. Each legitimate message is kept as an "item" to which all subsequent related messages can be attached. Volunteer librarians can log on to QRC at any time to make selections from the "Questions to be Answered" categories. Other available categories allow for various types of correspondence, patron feedback, and librarian discussion. QRC is being tested for its functionality in a variety of environments and has worked successfully in academic, public, and special libraries.

What conclusions can be drawn from our experience with electronically enhanced reference services? What will the future hold? Will the printed word as we know it vanish from our daily lives? Or, in the words of technologist Walt Crawford, "When will all existing library materials be converted to digital form?"[51] Of course, Crawford would not pose such a question if he didn't intend to answer it, and the title of his article, "Paper Persists: Why Physical Library Collections Still Matter," provides a big clue to the nature of his response: "Not in my lifetime, probably not in yours, and quite likely never. The task is too big and too expensive, and the reward keeps diminishing." Crawford's conclusions and his vision for the future probably mirror those of many working reference librarians:

- The future means both print and electronic communications.
- The future means both linear text and hypertext.
- The future means both mediation by librarians and direct access.
- The future means both collections and access.
- The future means a library that is both edifice and interface.[51]

At the close of the twentieth century, reference librarians can count upon a future that will continue to be filled with change; our future success will rest largely on our skills in dealing with that change. The Internet will continue to be both a delight and a frustration in receiving and answering the information needs of our patrons. Both print and electronic tools will continue to be used, although the emphasis (and the budgetary commitment) will continue to shift as well.

REFERENCE NOTES

1. Tenopir, C., and Ennis, L. "The Digital Reference World of Academic Libraries." *ONLINE* 1998. Available: <http://www.onlineinc.com/onlinemag/OL1998/tenopir7.html>. Accessed: 2 October 1998.

2. Dickens, C. *A Tale of Two Cities.* Book I, Chapter I. Organization for Community Networks Electronic Bookshelf. 22 November 1996. Available: <http://ofcn.org/cyber.serv/resource/bookshelf/1city10/book1/chapter01.html>. Accessed: 2 October 1998.

3. MEDLIB-L listserv. MEDLIB@listserv.acsu.buffalo.

4. Library, University of California, Berkeley. "Finding Information on the Internet: A Tutorial." 1997-1998. Available: <http://www.lib.berkeley.edu/TeachingLib/Guides/Internet/FindInfo.html>. Accessed: 2 October 1998.

5. Otto Lottes Health Sciences Library, University of Missouri. "Nothing But 'Net: An Internet Search Guide for Health Professionals." 19 May 1998. Available: <http://www.hsc.missouri.edu/library/docs/tutorial.html>. Accessed: 2 October 1998.

6. Committee on Institutional Cooperation. HealthWeb. 1 October 1998. Available: <http://www.healthweb.org>. Accessed: 2 October 1998.

7. Leita, C. Librarians' Index to the Internet. 27 September 1998. Available: <http://www.sunsite.berkeley.edu/InternetIndex>. Accessed: 2 October 1998.

8. University of Michigan, School of Information. Internet Public Library. 1995. Available: <http://www.ipl.org>. Accessed: 2 October 1998.

9. Balas, J. "The Importance of Mastering Search Engines." *Computers in Libraries* 18(May 1998): 42-4.

10. Lawrence, S., and Giles, C.L. "Searching the World Wide Web." *Science* 280 (3 April 1998): 98-100.

11. HotBot. Search Engine. 1994-1998. Wired Digital, Inc. Available: <http://www.hotbot.com>. Accessed: 2 October 1998.

12. AltaVista. Search Engine. 1995-1998. Digital Equipment Co. Available: <http://www.altavista.digital.com>. Accessed: 2 October 1998.

13. Excite. Search Engine. 1995-1998. Excite Inc. Available: <http://www.excite.com>. Accessed: 2 October 1998.

14. Infoseek. Search Engine. 1994-1998. Infoseek Corp. Available: <http://www.infoseek.com>. Accessed: 2 October 1998.

15. Lycos. Search Engine. 1998. Lycos, Inc. Available: <http://www.lycos.com>. Accessed: 2 October 1998.

16. Northern Light. Search Engine. 1997-1998. Northern Light Technology LLC. Available: <http://www.northernlight.com>. Accessed: 2 October 1998.

17. Ask Jeeves. Search Engine. 1998. Ask Jeeves, Inc. Available: <http://www.askjeeves.com>. Accessed: 2 October 1998.

18. MetaFind. Metasearch Engine. Available: <http://www.metasearch.com>. Accessed: 2 October 1998.

19. Inference Find. Metasearch Engine. 1995-1998. Inference Corp. Available: <http://www.infind.com>. Accessed: 2 October 1998.

20. Dogpile. Metasearch Engine. Available: <http://www.dogpile.com>. Accessed: 2 October 1998.

21. MetaCrawler. Metasearch Engine. 1997-1998. *Go@net, Inc.* Available: <http://www.metacrawler.com>. Accessed: 2 October 1998.

22. Search Engine Watch. 1996-1998. Mecklermedia Corp. Available: <http://www.searchenginewatch.com>. Accessed: 2 October 1998.

23. Notess, G. Search Engine Showdown. 1997-1998. Available: <http://imt.net/~notess/search>. Accessed: 2 October 1998.

24. Silberg, W.M.; Lundberg, G.D.; and Musacchio, R.A. "Assessing, Controlling, and Assuring the Quality of Medical Information on the Internet: *Caveant Lector et Viewor*—Let the Reader and Viewer Beware." *JAMA* 277(16 April 1997): 1244-5.

25. Health On the Net Foundation. 23 September 1998. Available: <http://www.hon.ch>. Accessed: 2 October 1998.

26. Health on the Net Foundation. "HONCode of Conduct for Medical and Health Websites." Version 1.6. April 1997. Available: <http://www.hon.ch/HONcode/Conduct.htm>. Accessed: 2 October 1998.

27. Health Information Technology Institute, Mitretek Systems, Inc. "White Paper: Criteria for Assessing the Quality of Health Information on the Internet." 14 October 1997. Available: <http://www.mitretek.org/hiti/showcase/documents.criteria.html>. Accessed: 2 October 1998.

28. Internet Healthcare Coalition. "Statement of Purpose." 1997. Available: <http://www.ihc.net>. Accessed: 2 October 1998.

29. Internet Healthcare Coalition. "Quality Healthcare Information on the 'Net '98: Delivering on the Promise, McLean, Virginia, October 5-6, 1998." Available: <http://www.virsci.com/ihc/conf.html>. Accessed: 2 October 1998.

30. Rettig, J. "Rettig on Reference." 1997, 1998. Available: <http://www.gale.com/gale/rettig/rettig.html>. Accessed: 2 October 1998.

31. Rettig, J. "Beyond Cool: Analog Models for Reviewing Digital Resources." *ONLINE* 1996. Available: <http://www.onlineinc.com/onlinemag/SeptOL/rettig9.html>. Accessed: 2 October 1998.

32. Anderson, P.F.; Allee, N.; Chung, J.; Westra, B.; and Lingle, V. "Comparison of Health Information Megasites." Poster session presented at the Annual Meeting, Medical Library Association, Philadelphia, PA, May 24-27, 1998. Available: <http://www.lib.umich.edu/megasite/>. Accessed: 2 October 1998.

33. McDermott, I.E., "The Internet Express: Virtual Reference for a Real Public." *Searcher* 1998. Available: <http://www.infotoday.com/searcher/apr98/story1.htm>. Accessed: 2 October 1998.

34. University of Southern California. Electronic Reference Shelf. 3 March 1998. Available: <http://www.usc.edu/Research/reference.html>. Accessed: 3 October 1998.

35. Purdue University Libraries. The Virtual Reference Desk. 25 June 1998. Available: <http://thorplus.lib.purdue.edu/reference/index.html>. Accessed: 2 October 1998.

36. Internet Public Library Reference Center. 27 April 1998. Available: <http://www.ipl.org/ref/>. Accessed: 2 October 1998.

37. *healthfinder*™. 28 April 1998. U.S. Department of Health and Human Services. Available: <http://www.healthfinder.gov>. Accessed: 2 October 1998.

38. National Library of Medicine. PubMed database. Available: <http://www.ncbi.nlm.nih.gov/PubMed/>. Accessed: 2 October 1998.

39. "Vice President Gore Launches Free MEDLINE." *NLM Newsline* 52(March-August 1997): 1-2, 11.

40. "Online Usage Statistics Smashed." *NLM Newsline* 53(January-March 1998): 1-2.

41. Rees, A.M., ed. *Consumer Health Information Source Book.* Fifth Edition. Phoenix, AZ: Oryx Press, 1998. p ix.

42. Warren, C. "Serving the Young and the Restless: Development of a Youth Health Collection in a Consumer Health Library." Paper presented at the Annual Meeting, Medical Library Association, Philadelphia, PA, May 24-27, 1998.

43. Earl, M.F.; Littleton, C.; Paden, S.; and Prichard, D. "Making a Difference: Determining the Impact of a Consumer Health Information Service on Participants' Attitudes, Health Care Decision Making, and Physician-Patient Communication." Paper presented at the Annual Meeting, Medical Library Association, Philadelphia, PA, May 24-27, 1998.

44. Bianchi, N.; Porter, D.; Bolkum, S.; Guitar, C.; Sekerak, R.; and McGowan, J. "VT CHIP: Health Care Information Consumers Define Need." Paper presented at the Annual Meeting, Medical Library Association, Philadelphia, PA, May 24-27, 1998.

45. "NLM Announces Plan to Increase Access to Health Information on the Internet: Thirty-Seven Public Libraries Chosen to Assist in Public Education Campaign." Press Release from the National Library of Medicine, July 28, 1998. Available: <http://www.nlm.nih.gov/news/press_releases/access.html>. Accessed: 2 October 1998.

46. MEDLINE*plus*. 22 October 1998. Available: <http://medlineplus.nlm.nih.gov/medlineplus/>. Accessed: 5 November 1998.

47. Fishman, D.L. "Managing the Virtual Reference Desk: How to Plan an Effective Reference E-Mail System." *Medical Reference Services Quarterly* 17(Spring 1998): 1-10.

48. Clintworth, W.A., and Nelson J.L. "Online Search Strategy Assistance: An Innovative Form of Distance Learning." Poster session presented at the Annual Meeting, Medical Library Association, Kansas City, MO, June 2-4, 1996.

49. Lagace. N., and McClennen, M. "Questions and Quirks: Managing an Internet-Based Distributed Reference Service." *Computers in Libraries* 18(February 1998): 22-4.

50. University of Michigan, School of Information. Internet Public Library. "Ask a Question Form." 5 June 1998. Available: <http://www.ipl.org/ref/QUE/RefFormQRC.html>. Accessed: 2 October 1998.

51. Crawford, W. "Paper Persists: Why Physical Library Collections Still Matter." *Online* 22(January 1998). Available: <http://www.onlineinc.com/onlinemag/OL98/crawford1.html>. Accessed: 2 October 1998.

Chapter 2

Natural Language and Beyond: Tips for Search Services

Eric P. Delozier

INTRODUCTION

It would not be misleading to argue that searching for information on the Internet is drastically different today than online searching of data aggregators was ten years ago. In fact, the days of adherence to strict Boolean logic and controlled vocabulary by database designers, programmers, and search intermediaries from a generation ago have been supplanted by systems utilizing underlying and complex techniques aimed at making the search process easier for the end user. Many of today's databases that maintain a record of content on the Internet employ methodologies such as natural language, relevance ranking, fuzzy logic, free text, and so on to locate relevant material without the need to learn complicated search formulations.

The most vocal opponents of natural language search systems are more often than not veteran search intermediaries, that is, librarians. A major complaint of natural language searching is that, oftentimes, a search engine returns too many irrelevant hits. Proponents, on the other hand, argue that traditional search interfaces are too difficult to maneuver. They argue that end users aren't interested in both high recall and precision. Rather, end users are mainly concerned with a few highly relevant hits (i.e., precision), without regard to what else might be available.

Depending on one's point of view, finding information on the Internet can be a simple process or an exercise in futility. This chapter attempts to offer some practical advice to maximize a searcher's time and efficiency. Specifically, it covers services that index Web pages, Usenet newsgroups, and electronic mailing lists. It excludes those services which dominated the Internet before the Web became so prevalent. Examples of these early services not covered in this chapter include Telnet directories, Archie, Veronica, and so on. Although interest in these legacy services has subsided in recent years, other publications[1-3] have covered them when they were prevalent.

CATEGORIES OF SEARCH FACILITIES

Whether termed indexes, databases, catalogs, engines, or directories, search services, as they are referred to in this article, as a rule, can be classified as engines, subject directories, or metasearch gateways. Each class of service is distinct, yet it is sometimes difficult to distinguish between the first two. For example, both subject directories and engines now permit a user to browse databases by way of a hierarchical listing of subject categories. Until recently, this feature was, for the most part, unique to the subject directories.

Engines

Commonly called spiders, crawlers, or robots, these services are characterized by their ability to build a database without a human intermediary. Although humans may write the programs that allow engines to build a database, the actual process of locating content and building the database is accomplished without intervention. Robots continuously visit and revisit content providers in search of material that should be added, changed, or deleted from their massive databases. While doing so, they adhere to strict procedures designed to prevent overwhelming the resources of the visited server. The largest of all search services, in terms of database size, is HotBot (http://www.hotbot.com/). Other popular search engines with established reputations include Excite (http://www.excite.com/), AltaVista (http://altavista.digital.com/), Infoseek (http://www.infoseek.com/), Lycos (http://www.lycos.com/), Northern Light (http://www.

northernlight.com/), and WebCrawler (http:// www.webcrawler.com/). Medical World Search (http://www.mwsearch.com/) combines a search engine with the Unified Medical Language System (UMLS) thesaurus that maps user input to appropriate indexing terms.

Subject Directories

Whereas engines aren't totally dependent upon human intervention, directories, on the other hand, are. Directory databases are built by humans, often librarians, who analyze Web pages for inclusion or exclusion. Directories typically allow a user to browse, without initially having to enter a keyword, by way of broad categories often arranged hierarchically. Similar to pure engines, they also allow a user to search by keyword. Their databases are typically smaller than engines, since the presence of human intervention adds time to the building process. Content is usually acquired using electronic forms completed by the entity offering Web pages or via promotion services such as Submit It! (http://www.submit-it.com/). Better-known subject directories include Yahoo! (http://www.yahoo.com), Galaxy (http://www.einet.net/galaxy.html), Internet Public Library (http://ipl.si.umich.edu/), and Argus Clearinghouse (http://www.clearinghouse.net/). Also included in this category are subject-specific directories. Examples of these include HealthWeb (http://www.healthweb.org/), Medical Matrix (http://www.medmatrix.org/), MedWeb (http://www.gen.emory.edu/ medweb/ medweb.html), NOAH (http://noah.cuny.edu/), Combined Health Information Database (http://chid.nih.gov/), healthfinder (http://www.healthfinder.gov/), and CliniWeb (http://www.ohsu.edu/ cliniweb/). CliniWeb is an experimental directory that is restricted to clinical content and browseable by Medical Subject Heading (MeSH).

Metasearch Gateways

Metasearch gateways are characterized by their ability to simultaneously or individually query search engines using a consistent form. They are distinguished by the fact that they don't build and index content. Hence, they don't have any database to maintain. Rather, they submit search requests to multiple services, then compile and display the results, usually on one page, to the user. Meta-search gateways are valuable for rare topics, since they offer a user the convenience of submitting one search to many engines. This thereby saves the user time, since he or she doesn't have to retype the same query individually and repeatedly to each service. The downside to metasearch gateways is that they offer less functionality than individual services. Because individual search services handle more complex queries in their own unique manner, metasearch gateways normally accept simple queries then convert them to a common format shared by the collective group. Those which query multiple engines simultaneously include MetaCrawler (http://www.metacrawler.com/), Dogpile (http://www.dogpile.com/), Inference Find (http://www.infind.com/), Internet Sleuth (http://www.isleuth.com/), MetaFind (http://www.metafind.com/), and Mamma (http://www.mamma.com/).

GETTING STARTED

Learn the Landscape

Early Internet search applications focused on the delivery mechanism used to make the information available. Long before the Web became popular, other delivery mechanisms such as e-mail, file transfer protocol (FTP), Telnet, Usenet, and, later, Gopher, were utilized as information transfer agents, with little or no gateway from one to another. For example, Archie was developed as a tool to find files available via FTP only. Hence, a user could not utilize Archie to discover if anyone posted a message to a Usenet news-group on Creutzfeldt-Jakob disease. On the other hand, many Web-based search services now allow a user to specify what information service he or she wants the information to originate from. As Figure 2.1 illustrates, it is now possible to restrict a search in Yahoo! to one of several delivery mechanisms. Infoseek allows the user to search not only the Web and Usenet but also specialized news (PR Newswire, Business Wire, and Reuters) and company information (Hoover's Company Profiles) sources (see Figure 2.2).

FIGURE 2.1. Yahoo! Search Engine Home Page

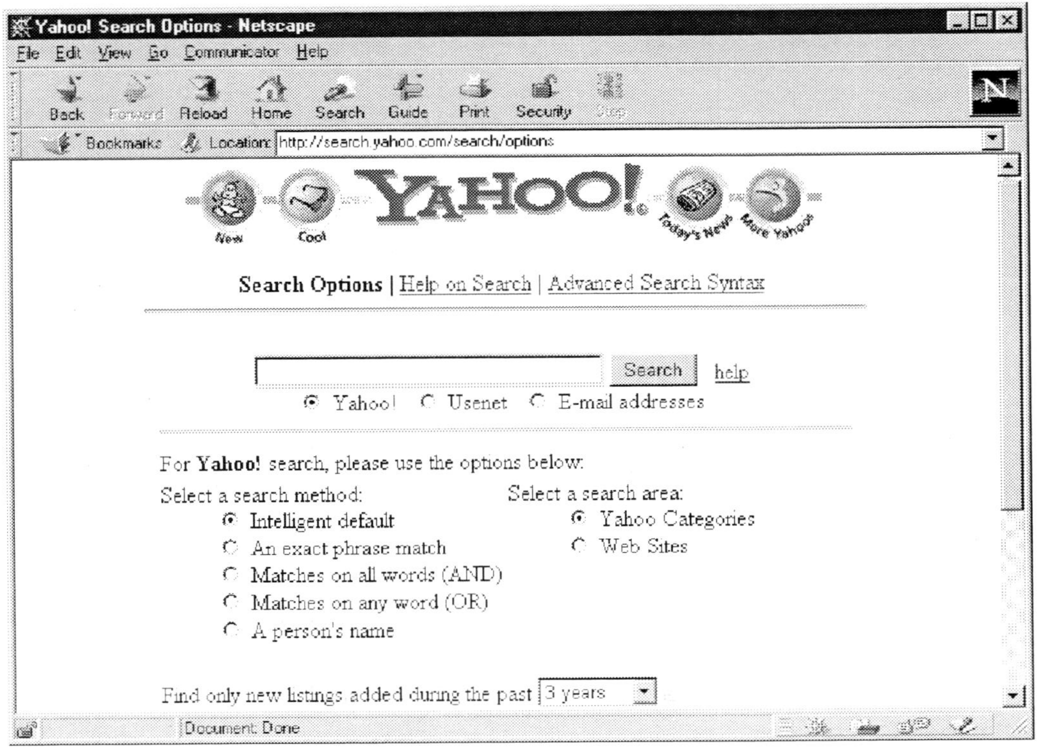

Yahoo! Search Options - Netscape

File Edit View Go Communicator Help

Back Forward Reload Home Search Guide Print Security Stop

Bookmarks Location: http://search.yahoo.com/search/options

YAHOO!

Today's News   More Yahoo!

Search Options | Help on Search | Advanced Search Syntax

Search   help

For **Yahoo!** search, please use the options below.

Select a search method: Select a search area:
○ Intelligent default   ⊙ Yahoo Categories
○ An exact phrase match   ○ Web Sites
○ Matches on all words (AND)
○ Matches on any word (OR)
○ A person's name

⊙ Yahoo!   ○ Usenet   ○ E-mail addresses

Find only new listings added during the past 3 years ▼

Document: Done

17

FIGURE 2.2. Infoseek Search Engine Home Page

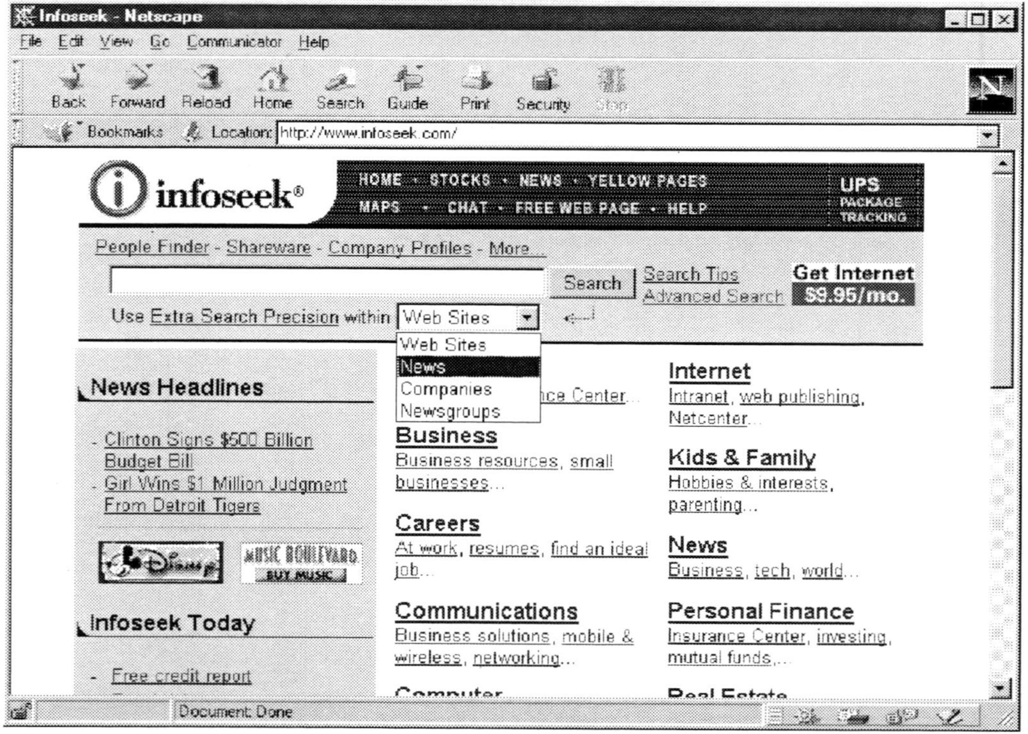

Browsing

An incredible amount of health information on the Web is targeted to both consumers and health professionals. The Web is saturated with so much information that simply getting started can be overwhelming to the user. It is generally advisable to begin by browsing and getting comfortable with those services which have already cataloged information. Veteran searchers generally begin by familiarizing themselves with one of the specialized medical or health subject directories. Yahoo! Health Information: Web Directories (http://dir.yahoo.com/Health/Web_Directories/) included almost forty entries at the time this chapter was written. Among those listed is the Hardin Meta Directory of Internet Health Sources (http://www.lib.uiowa.edu/hardin/md/), a directory of directories arranged by medical specialty. The Hardin Meta Directory also includes the Comprehensive Health and Medical Index (http://www.lib.uiowa.edu/hardin/md/idx.html), which includes a listing of those directories with established and reliable track records for providing reliable information sources.

The previous discussion of browsing concentrated on, for the most part, utilizing sources for browsing Web pages. However, other delivery mechanisms in addition to the Web also lend themselves to browsing. Group discussions in the form of electronic mailing lists and Usenet newsgroups allow users to communicate with others in a group environment.

Usenet newsgroups resemble electronic bulletin boards where an individual can post information that others can read at their convenience. Groups are categorized into broad categories, such as science, computers, society, recreation, and so on. Deja News (http://www.dejanews.com/) is a unique service that extracts messages from their original groups and reclassifies them into more meaningful categories. Under Health, it includes a broad range of topics such as Children's Health, Diseases and Disorders, Women's Health, and so on.

Group discussions aren't limited to Usenet, however. Many individuals regularly receive mass mailings electronically from special-interest groups. Receipt of mail depends upon whether a user is a subscriber to the list. These mailing lists utilize software such as LISTSERV, Majordomo, or Listprocessor to manage subscribers and mailings. Although mailing list messages aren't generally readable unless a user is a subscriber, some innovative directories do make it easier to locate and subscribe to a list of interest. Two that offer extensive inventories with browsing features are Tile.net (http://tile.net/lists/) and Publicly Accessible Mailing Lists (http://www.neosoft.com/internet/paml/).

BEYOND NATURAL LANGUAGE

Virtually all Internet search services initially present the user with a basic form that encourages simplicity. The user enters a query and the service returns a list of pages based on a number of strategies. Some services make use of sophisticated statistical algorithms or "fuzzy logic." Others automatically combine the terms and return a list matching any word entered, that is, implied "or." There are those which even return a list in which all terms are present, that is, implied "and."

The ensuing discussion will deal with exploiting the more advanced features of search services. Most, if not all, the major engines and directories allow the user to go beyond the simple interface and construct rather sophisticated search statements that make use of Boolean and positional operators in addition to field searching. These features are normally found by referring to a service's advanced options or help pages.

Discovering the peculiarities of various search services is not as difficult as it may appear. Fortunately, others have taken steps to document and chart many features beyond natural language that services support. *Power Searching for Anyone* (http://www.searchenginewatch.com/facts/powersearch.html) by Danny Sullivan and the *Search Engine Comparison Chart* (http://www.kcpl.lib.mo.us/search/chart.htm) from the Kansas City Public Library both list advanced searching features and how they are implemented on various search services. Susan Feldman, in an article that reviews the trends and challenges of search services, also includes a feature comparison chart.[4]

Applying Operators

Finding All Terms

Use of the Boolean "and" operator is generally supported by most search services through a combination of any one or all of the following methods: implied, menus (e.g., pull-down or radio buttons), a special symbol such as a plus sign (+), or by literally typing "and" as part of the search statement. If a service requires the use of +, it is important to remember that all terms must be preceded by the symbol. Therefore, a properly constructed statement that returns all pages containing both Viagra and women would appear as *+viagra +women*. A statement that includes the symbol before only one word (i.e., *+viagra women*) implies the presence of Viagra with or without women.

Finding Any Terms

As with Boolean "and," "or" is supported by any one or all of numerous methods. Included among these methods are implied, menus, or typing "or" as part of the statement. It is generally advisable to qualify a search statement with parentheses and another Boolean operator when searching for any one or another word or both. Therefore, a properly constructed statement that requires methotrexate and either eczema or psoriasis would appear as *(eczema or psoriasis) +methotrexate*. The same statement could also be entered correctly as *(eczema or psoriasis) and methotrexate*.

Excluding Terms

A search service's support of exclusion is usually implemented through menus, literal inclusion, or a symbol such as a minus sign (−). As a rule, some action must be taken by the user to exclude a term from a search statement. Hence, there is no implied "not." When using a symbol to indicate exclusion, it is important to point out that the character must precede the word; otherwise, the search service will interpret the term's presence as optional or mandatory, depending on how the engine interprets the absence of an operator. An acceptable example of a search statement utilizing the minus sign to include the terms hair and finasteride but not minoxidil would be entered as *+hair +finasteride −minoxidil*. The same statement could also be properly entered as *(hair and finasteride) not minoxidil*. Yet a third way to construct the previous statement is *(hair and finasteride) and not minoxidil*. It is therefore strongly advised that users carefully observe a service's requirement for specifying exclusion.

Phrase Searching

Virtually all search services will return a list of documents where two or more words appear in exact order. This feature is almost universally implemented by surrounding the search statement phrase with quotation marks (e.g., *"quinacrine sterilization"*). Many services also offer phrase searching by allowing the user to choose a menu item on the same page that a user enters the search statement. Excite and HotBot support either method.

Proximity

A variation on phrase searching is the ability to locate documents where two or more words appear, but with a certain number of other terms or characters in between. "Near" is the standard operator for proximity searching for those services which offer the feature, although its semantics varies. As an example, consider the following search statement: *quinacrine near sterilization*. In the preceding example, AltaVista returns documents where a maximum of ten words appears between quinacrine and sterilization. Lycos, on the other hand, defaults to twenty-five words.

Lycos also provides additional and extensive proximity features. Some variations on the previous search statement in Lycos include *quinacrine far sterilization* (greater than twenty-five words between), *quinacrine adj sterilization* (no words between and any order), *quinacrine before sterilization* (any number of words between and exact order). Lycos also allows a user to specify the number and order of intervening words. Order is specified by preceding the operator with the letter O, while the maximum number of intervening words is designated by appending a forward slash (/) then a number. A search statement that returns all documents in Lycos where quinacrine appears before sterilization and with no more than five intervening words would be entered as *quinacrine Onear/5 sterilization*.

Wildcards

Whether termed wildcard, stem, or truncation, this feature is supported by virtually all services. The most common method is to append or precede the term with an asterisk (*).

FIELD SEARCHING

At first glance, documents on the Web do not seem to resemble traditional types of print-based publications, whose physical descriptions provide structure and organization to bibliographic catalogs and electronic databases. However, a closer examination reveals that Web pages do indeed contain discreet components. These components become searchable fields for those search services which choose to implement them as such. The ensuing discussion will briefly describe the four components commonly used for field searching: title, URL (uniform resource locator), body, and link. Hock provides a more thorough discussion, including a useful chart that lists features and required syntax for field searching of various services.[5]

Title

The document title is the first of perhaps two fields that offers some resemblance to its bibliographic counterparts. The title is actually an HTML (hypertext markup language) tag and subset of the document header. A user sees it on the title bar of the browser displaying the document. The bar, the uppermost part of an application's display, usually includes the browser name and title of the opened document. It's worth noting that a title can also appear on the same page as the body (see the following subsection), provided the content author chooses to do so. The source HTML tag that contains the title can be viewed with most Web browsers. AltaVista, Yahoo!, and Infoseek support title searching with the *title:* prefix (e.g., *title:"atkins diet"*). HotBot, on the other hand, utilizes menus.

Body

Besides the title, the body of a Web-based document is the second component that bears some bibliographic resemblance. Normally, it isn't necessary to qualify a search statement because virtually all search services default to the document text or title. Services such as Infoseek and Lycos, which offer advanced search options via menus that specify the entire document, will perform a full-text search. This type of search naturally is more costly in terms of computer resources and, often, relevancy. Therefore, it should be avoided unless the topic is rare.

Uniform Resource Locator

A third item commonly used for field searching is composed of elements that make up the uniform resource locator (URL), or page address. When broken down, the URL contains an address, a directory path, and a file name, for example, <http://cancernet.nci.nih.gov/clinpdq/therapy.html>. In this example, the address (cancernet.nci.nih.gov), directory path (clinpdq), and file name (therapy.html) are delineated with a forward slash (/). Searching usually involves prefixing a search statement with a keyword, for example, *url:nci.nih.gov and ti:prostate*. The preceding example entered in AltaVista returns all documents from the National Cancer Institute containing the word prostate in the title.

Citation Searching

Infoseek, AltaVista, and HotBot all offer a feature that allows a user to retrieve a list of documents that link to or cite a specified URL. Analogous to citation searching of bibliographic databases for which the Institute for Scientific Information is known, link can be useful for measuring the value of a Web site. Consider the reduced carbohydrate weight loss program, the Atkins Diet (http://www.atkinscenter.com/), which has its share of both defenders and critics. A user can conduct a link search, for example, *link: www.atkinscenter. com*, in Infoseek and retrieve a list of documents that refers to Dr. Atkins' Web pages. Link searching is also a useful tool for Webmasters who want to evaluate the merit of their content by determining who points to their pages.

WORDS OF WISDOM

Searching the Internet for information is often a paradox. The information is probably available; however, with so many options at one's disposal, the experience can be frustrating. With so many competing search services, the most difficult part of the process is often deciding where to start. The following tips are generalized, intending to encompass strategies that the reader can apply to any search service, whether it be an engine, directory, or metasearch engine.

Become Acquainted with More Than One Search Service

No Internet search service exhaustively indexes the Internet. A recent study in *Science* concluded that search services cover, at most, approximately one third of what is available to them.[6] Notess recommends that a comprehensive search of the Web should encompass the four largest services (HotBot, AltaVista, Infoseek, and Excite).[7]

Read Search Service Documentation

There is no industry standard, for example, Z39.50, to which search services must adhere. A user therefore cannot assume that the syntax for one service is the same as for another. All services provide online documentation that covers all features.

Exploit Boolean and Field Searches

The debate over natural language versus Boolean searching will continue. In an effort to satisfy both sides of the issue and to remain competitive, search services will continue to support both. Although natural language often returns relevant pages, Boolean searching is required for comprehensiveness.

Use Metasearch Engines with Caution

It is worth noting that although metasearch gateways may save users time by repeating the same search across multiple services, they have limitations. Metasearch services will sometimes utilize a common denominator so that one search statement will work across multiple indexes. This means that Boolean or field statements may be converted to natural language to work in more than one service.

Second, not all search services are accessible to metasearch gateways. Apparently, none of them can search Northern Light and only a few can reach HotBot. Greg Notess, in a more thorough critique (http://imt.net/~notess/search/multip.html) of metasearch gateways, covers the topic in greater detail.

REFERENCE NOTES

1. Howe, W., and Tillman, H.N. "Searching on the Internet," in *Internet Tools of the Profession*, edited by H.N. Tillman. Washington, DC: Special Libraries Association, 1995, 9-53.

2. Gilster, P. *Finding It on the Internet: The Essential Guide to Archie, Veronica, Gopher, WAIS, WWW (Including Mosaic), and Other Search and Browsing Tools.* New York: Wiley, 1994.

3. Delozier, E.P. "Strategies for Finding Information on the Internet: Getting Started with Archie, Gopher, WWW, and WAIS." *Medical Reference Services Quarterly* 15(Summer 1996):61-5.

4. Feldman, S. "Web Service Services in 1998: Trends and Challenges." *Searcher* 6(June 1998):29-39.

5. Hock, R. "How to Do Field Searching in Web Search Engines: A Field Trip." *Online* 22(May/June 1998):19-22.

6. Lawrence, S., and Giles, C.L. "Searching the World Wide Web." *Science* 280(April 3, 1998):98-100.

7. Notess, G.R. "On the Net. Measuring the Size of Internet Databases." *Database* 20(October/November 1997):69-70.

Chapter 3

Megasites for Health Care Information

Cindy A. Gruwell
Scott Marsalis

INTRODUCTION

What, you may ask, is a "megasite," and how can megasites help one to locate quality health care information? As the good witch Glinda says, "it's always best to start at the beginning," so let's begin by looking at the term itself. The World Wide Web is made up of a myriad "sites," each of which contains multiple layers, or "pages." Although these pages and sites have real and intellectual finiteness, they are interconnected (linked) into the wondrous, and often over-whelming, weave of the Web. One locates the nuggets of useful information by utilizing search engines or by following links that someone has constructed from his or her own site. The other part of our word is the prefix "mega," which is technically defined as meaning one million.[1] So, a "megawatt" is a million watts, and a megabyte is a million bytes. However, "mega" has evolved in the vernacular to mean simply "huge." The Mall of America is the megamall, and a hot summer movie is declared a megahit. The Internet, land of hyperbole, has adopted the latter meaning, and so we refer to sites containing large amounts of information and links as a megasite. The Internet is also a land of anarchy, riddled with battles fought with buzzwords and mega-bucks, so we also have the related (and sometimes interchangeable) term "metasite." Our preference is to use the term metasite to refer to those sites primarily made up of links to other sites, with little added intellectual value beyond the construction and organization of the links. Although some of the sites we will be discussing arguably fit into that definition, most move beyond that, acting as a filter to gather the best sites, organizing and annotating them, and usually adding documents of their own. Some megasites discussed fit into the other end of the spectrum, containing few links, but gathering, organizing, and mounting on their site quality health care information. We will be including sites that fit along the range of these definitions, but all are "mega" in that they address a broad range of health-related topics.

"Very nice, Glinda," you say, "but exactly what does this have to do with finding quality health care information?" Megasites act as a way to skip right to the good stuff. We've all experienced the frustration of using multiple search engines to look for relevant information, only to be faced with wading through pages of irrelevant "matches" to find a few good sites. Even more frustrating is trying to find that good site you know is out there, but for some reason isn't being retrieved by any of the popular engines. With megasites, you get to draw on the hard work of qualified professionals who have done the searching, evaluating, and compiling for you (find information on breast cancer without having to wade through pages of soft porn!). The megasites also provide one-site access to a breadth of information. The Web is an evolving entity, and megasites can help bring order to the chaos. Change may include relocation of a site to another URL (uniform resource locator) or merely a different appearance or organization of a site. A good megasite keeps on top of the changes, updating its links regularly. Another benefit of megasites is their frequent inclusion of sources a search engine can't pull up, which may even be better than a print counterpart. For example, Mayo Health Oasis's medical glossary not only provides concise definitions but also hyperlinked cross-references and an audio pronunciation guide.

Now that we've sold you on the benefits of megasites, we should discuss some of the qualities to look for in a good site. Jim Kapoun of Southwest State University suggests applying the same criteria in evaluating Web sites as in selecting print references, which he concisely expresses as "Accuracy, Authority, Objectivity, Currency and Coverage."[2] In health care, information accuracy is especially critical, and a lot of unsubstantiated and fraudulent claims are published on the Internet. The Health On the Net Foundation (HON) is a nonprofit international organization dedicated to promoting quality health care information on the Internet and helping to realize the

Internet's potential as a valuable medical information resource. Although displaying the HON icon is testament to a site's quality, a lot of excellent sites do not display it. Nevertheless, the HON Principles and Code of Conduct further guide one in evaluating health information sites. We won't include the full principles here (they are available on the HON Web site, <http://www.hon.ch>), but we've incorporated many of the ideas into the following guidelines.

When evaluating a site, a good first step is to look at the Web address as well as the identified sponsors of the site. The host's suffix will help identify whether it is an educational (.edu), government (.gov), nonprofit (.org), or commercial (.com) site; however, other countries have their own suffixes, and the suffix may be misleading. A page with an .edu address may be the product of a student or alum and not officially affiliated with the educational institution at all. The Virtual Hospital, a product of the University of Iowa, has a .org address. A good site will clearly identify who the sponsors are and provide information for contacting at least the Webmaster, if not the chief editors as well. Individual authors and editors should also be identified, along with their qualifications, to aid in judging the authority and accuracy of the site's contents.

Objectivity is arguably impossible, so it pays to be mindful of all the degrees of bias of a site. Some other things to keep in mind—a site that accepts advertising should clearly identify copy as such, as well as prominently posting its policies for accepting advertisers or sponsors. Remember to look at the credentials of the authors and editors. A medical doctor (MD), doctor of chiropractic (DC), and doctor of osteopathy (DO) will each have his or her own biases. A degreed librarian will bring different skills and biases to a site than will an MD. Any textual information should have its creation date clearly identified. Good sites also identify areas newly updated and have a minimum of obsolete links. The intended audience of a site should be identified, and the information should be appropriate to that audience. With a megasite, you'll want to see that the site addresses a range of topics: Are there a good number of links? Are the links made to appropriate sites, and are they well organized and annotated? Quality sites, especially those aimed at patients, should include a statement that the information is not intended as a replacement for the advice of a professional physician and that the patient should discuss any concerns with his or her provider, especially before changing or undertaking any new treatments or therapies. Finally, a good megasite should be designed so that it can be easily and quickly navigated. A site with extraneous bells and whistles may have been fun to design, but also unusable to those with slower modems or earlier browser versions.

All that said, what follows is a highly annotated list of some of the best megasites we have seen. Each is unique and possesses individual qualities that may influence how often you do or do not use a site. We've broken the sites into three general categories: those intended for patients or other consumers; those sites which are "information intensive," containing primarily information and a minimum of links; and those intended primarily for medical professionals. Of course, these divisions are rather artificial, and many of the sites could arguably be placed in multiple sections, but we hope they will help you in selecting your favorites.

CONSUMER HEALTH SITES

Note: Please also see Chapter 6, "Consumer Health Information on the Internet," for a broader discussion on this topic.

One of the more challenging tasks in health sciences librarianship is finding quality information for patrons who do not have the education to effectively comprehend the more technical literature and resources such as MEDLINE or to critically sort through the nontechnical health information that proliferates on the Internet. Although many excellent sites, such as that of the American Cancer Society, provide reputable information on individual diseases, disorders, or groups of diseases, the following megasites cover a broad range of health topics, serving as good starting points for finding quality information in easily understood language.

New York Online Access to Health (NOAH) <http://www.noah.cuny.edu>

NOAH is the result of a 1995 U.S. Department of Commerce National Telecommunications and Information Administration grant to the City University of New York, the Metropolitan Library Council, the New York Academy of Medicine, and the New York Public Library. Since then, other partners have joined, allowing the site to grow into a premier source for online health information for consumers. NOAH's uniqueness lies in its philosophy of outreach to consumers of socioeconomic classes traditionally underserved by health information sources, providing access through 100 partner libraries in New York's public library systems and on CUNY campuses, as well as to the global community via the Web. Because many of the traditionally underserved groups also are Spanish speaking, NOAH has broadened its commitment by acting as a bilingual site, presenting information in Spanish as well as in English.

NOAH provides full-text consumer health information and links to other quality sites via over forty topical pages ranging from AIDS, cancer, and other diseases to pages focusing on healthy living, sexuality, or nutrition. These specialized pages are reached via a well-laid-out "Health Topics" page, which divides the pages into two sections, "Health Topics" and "Resources." The latter consists of links to other sites, arranged topically into the following categories: New York City, State, and Regional Hospitals, HMOs, and Hospices; New York City County Resources; Patients Rights and Resources and Physician Information; Support Groups; Statistics; and Other Internet Resources. This page is compact, allowing users with limited screen size and modem speeds to utilize the site without waiting for endless graphics to load or forever scrolling up and down a long list. A simple box with links to all the areas of the site appears at the top and bottom of each NOAH screen, further simplifying and expediting navigation. New pages are highlighted, as are pages updated in the past month. The "What's New" page identifies areas updated or added in the past month, with several past months' records retained as well. The "Search by Word" page allows one to search using an Excite search engine, which searches only words contained in documents on the NOAH site, or a Harvest engine, which also searches NOAH's off-site links.

NOAH is very up-front in identifying the partners who fund the site, as well as in giving information on the contributing editors, all of whom, with one exception, are professional librarians (the latter being a journalist and author specializing in medical and health information). Biographical information on the editors is available, and on each page, the responsible author/editor is prominently identified. One noteworthy page is dedicated to teaching searchers how to evaluate for themselves the quality and biases of health information on the Web. Because its sponsors fund the site, advertising is not accepted.

Although NOAH does include a good deal of New York-specific information, its scope is much broader, making it useful to a global user group. Furthermore, by offering much of the information on the site in both Spanish and English, this megasite bridges a gap in the consumer health information arena.

Health Oasis: Mayo Clinic
<http://www.mayohealth.org>

A team of Mayo Clinic physicians, scientists, writers, and educators produces Mayo Health Oasis. Its primary content is informational texts; therefore, links to other sites, although significant, are not its main focus. The site is geared toward patients and other consumers and includes significant information on "wellness" topics such as nutrition and exercise. It addresses more controversial topics, such as the medicinal use of St. John's Wort, in a balanced, responsible manner. Health Oasis's design and content is similar to a high-quality print magazine, and although it is a good resource when looking for specific information, it is also a fascinating and informative site to visit regularly.

The Mayo Clinic is a household name, with an international reputation for quality, and Mayo Health Oasis maintains the institution's high standards of excellence. It subscribes to the Health On the Net (HON) principles for quality health information on the Internet, displaying the HON Code icon and link to that organization's site. The Health Oasis does accept advertising; however, it prominently posts its policy for including such advertisement and is careful to separate the advertisements from its editorial content. Although the site is well designed, with a minimum of extraneous graphics, the advertisements, unfortunately, are largely graphical, often animated, and can cause pages to load at a snail's pace when operating at a lower baud rate. Another commercial aspect of the site derives from the fact that Mayo publishes several reference texts, such as the *Mayo Clinic Family Health Book*, and these are available for purchase from the site.

Mayo Health Oasis's real strength is in providing solid information on current topics of interest. The site is updated every weekday, and new additions are highlighted on the home page. You can also subscribe to "HouseCall," a free, electronic weekly bulletin sent to your e-mail address notifying you of new additions to the site. The additions to Health Oasis are often timely, addressing new studies and media stories or providing updates on new drugs and treatments. The Headline Watch section gives brief introductions to longer documents elsewhere on the site, as well as highlighting the latest health news. The site is highly "interactive," providing health quizzes on topics such as "Do You Have Hay Fever?" and "Diabetes, Are You at Risk?" There is an Ask Mayo section where you can submit questions or read through previous topics. These questions and answers are not an attempt at practicing virtual medicine, but rather address topics such as "What Are Acoustic Tumors?" or "What's the Difference Between Cocoa and Chocolate, and What Is Carob?" The answers, written by a Mayo staff physician or dietitian, not only inform, but also link the reader to related documents and pages on the site. The writing on the site, as a whole, is quite good, appropriate to a lay audience, yet including enough technical details to aid the patient in understanding and communicating with his or her physician.

Mayo Health Oasis, however, is more than just an electronic popular health journal; it is a virtual library providing reference texts and links to other sites. One strength is its use of the capabilities of the Internet to enhance the value of the information. For example, if you have a sound card on your computer, the medical glossary not only defines medical terms, it also plays an audio file of the correct pronunciation. The high quality of the site, its readability, and the reputation associated with the Mayo name all recommend it as a megasite worth visiting.

WellnessWeb
<http://www.wellweb.com>

WellnessWeb offers few links to other sites; however, it is included in this chapter because of its coverage of a broad range of health topics and its unique patient-centered philosophy. It includes information on both conventional medicine and alternative/complementary medicine, and the site is easy to navigate due to its simple and concise layout.

WellnessWeb is subtitled "The Patient's Network," and its focus is information for patients and other consumers. This philosophy is notably evident in the site's presentation of the credentials of the editorial board. The editors are a diverse mix of medical professionals and professionals from medical technology companies or nonallied fields. Although all have extensive professional qualifications, they are first identified as "patient" or "parent of patient." For example, Dr. Richard Berkowitz is listed as "Prostate Cancer Patient/Professional Oversight—Richard is a graduate of Harvard College and Tufts Medical School; retired Professor Emeritus of the Temple University Medical School; and an extremely well informed patient of prostate cancer."[3] This patient orientation pervades the site, reflecting a commitment to providing information that is authoritative and accurate, but also comprehensible, to patients.

WellnessWeb subscribes to the HON principles for quality health information on the Internet, and although in some ways it seems to fall short, for the most part, it does maintain HON's high standards. The site does utilize "cookies," so confidentiality may be compromised. The "Grassroots" and "Online Bookstore" both feature user-submitted entries, and the identity and qualifications of the submitter are not always clear, so much caution must be used with information gleaned from these areas. The book reviews at the Online Bookstore are frequently submitted by the author and, thus, are especially subjective. The Bookstore page has an arrangement with Amazon.com, the Internet superbookstore, allowing users to purchase books reviewed on the site through Amazon.com, with part of the profits returned to WellnessWeb.

The site is generally easy to navigate, with a minimum of graphics and a fairly intuitive layout. From the home screen, the user can choose Conventional Medicine, Alternative/Complementary Medicine, Nutrition and Fitness, Calendar of Events, What's New, and a link for e-mailing the site. A phone number for contacting the editors is prominently displayed on the home page, although the date of the latest revision is not. Within the site, one can easily link to related pages, and, occasionally, appropriate links are made to pages outside WellnessWeb. Individual essays are attributed and often include references; however, they are not always dated. At the top of each section, there is a "What's New" column with the latest information, often covering recent studies and identifying the source. The introduction, although difficult to find buried in the What's New section, has a good discussion of WellnessWeb's mission, guidelines for therapy inclusions, and a basic discussion of when and why alternative therapies are included. The introduction to the section on alternative/complementary medicine has a more complete discussion of holistic approaches, regulation of supplements versus medicines, the veracity of double-blind studies, and other topics necessary for critically using health information. The section also covers the latest studies (with citations), media stories, fads, books, and "quackery" in a critical, balanced manner, as well as incorporating user comments and discussions. The section on conventional medicine is similarly laid out, with a section covering current news as well as essays on specific diseases and syndromes.

Although WellnessWeb is not without its faults, generally it is a high-quality site with good information on both conventional and complementary therapies. It maintains a strong patient orientation, without desolving into a site for the latest unsubstantiated therapy or total adherence to the American Medical Association (AMA) party line. As with all health information on the Web, the user needs to read the information offered critically, yet it is a good source covering a broader range of therapies and topics than other sites.

INFORMATION-INTENSIVE SITES

For our purposes, an information-intensive site is one that includes a wide variety of information in a variety of forms, as well as having organized links in a series of subject areas. Although no two megasites are exactly alike, they do have some commonalities that bring them together under this category. They all include actual documents, pamphlets, press releases, news stories, and so forth. In addition, each site is organized into sections contained within the site that pull together a myriad of information under a number of subject headings. These are all medical in nature and include consumer topics, general information, and professional subjects.

The following four Web sites reviewed are information intensive in nature. Each has similar, and yet unique, properties that will be discussed, along with some of the specific qualities, general navigation aspects, production of information, advertising, privacy, and other particulars of each site. It is hoped that the descriptions will provide insight into each megasite's usefulness and ability to provide information for general and, in some cases, specialized needs.

Achoo: Healthcare Online
<http://www.achoo.com>

Achoo: Healthcare Online is an Internet health care directory aimed at consumers, professionals, and people involved in the business of health care. Achoo is owned and managed by MNI Systems Corporation, which specializes in a variety of Internet and health care areas. Information is well organized in several sections. A disclaimer runs on the page indicating that the medical information provided on the site is for educational purposes only. Advertising is also allowed, with instructions for inclusion noted on the front page.

This site is fairly easy to use. Because of the overall organization into subject areas, all that is necessary is to point and click. The main menu and highlights area accentuates the basic aspects of the site. In addition, there is a search feature at the bottom of the page that allows full-text searching of the complete Web site.

This site has several unique features. These include Headline News, a comprehensive Internet health care news service; Reference/Resources, a variety of Internet resource materials covering numerous subjects; and Coming Features, a place where you can make comments and suggestions for upcoming features on the site.

Although Achoo provides a vast amount of information that seems up to date, there is a problem in verifying the currency. Unless one goes into some of the very specific sites, such as Headline News, which dates its news releases, there is no true date stamp. There is a yearly copyright designator, but this in no way replaces a revised or creation date that should be present at the bottom of the page. Aside from this flaw, Achoo does serve users well with interesting and useful information. In addition, the many links that are provided serve to connect consumers, professionals, and people in the business of health care to useful and relevant information.

Healthfinder ™
\<http://www.healthfinder.com>

Developed by the Department of Health and Human Services and several other governmental agencies, healthfinder is considered a "gateway" for a variety of consumer health and human services information. This site strives to provide current and reliable information to the public at large by providing links to selected publications, clearinghouses, databases, support/self-help groups, Web sites, and so on. Unlike some Web sites, healthfinder is not only well organized but also has an extremely easy-to-use subject listing. Sections include Hot Topics, News, Smart Choices, More Tools, Just for You, and About Us. There is substantial information available about the selection process as well as areas such as awards, contributing agencies, and feedback. Web site contact information exists on the About Us page. A nice plus is that healthfinder doesn't have advertising or annoying cookies that attempt to record your personal information.

Although the information is up to date, as noted in individual pages, the general pages with site links are not copyright dated, nor do they note updates or revisions. There is mention of updating on the About Us page; however, there seems to be no attempt to inform the public about the overall currency of the site.

Healthfinder is link driven; no search engine exists. Still, the extensive and informative subject listings prove easy to use. Unique features include links to a variety of resources that contain fully functional databases, full-text brochures, press releases, and so on. It is fairly quick to respond to requests, without the complexity of Java to slow it down. When all is said and done, healthfinder provides a wealth of information through its many links to the world.

HealthAtoZ: The Search Engine for Health and Medicine
\<http://www.healthatoz.com>

HealthAtoZ is a specialized search engine that covers various aspects of the health and medical community. This Web site is intended for both consumers and professionals, with plenty of information that is appropriate to both groups. Produced by medical professionals, with doctors and nurses writing the articles, HealthAtoZ attempts to provide a variety of articles, annotated links, and the ability to directly search MEDLINE.

Be aware that in order to make use of this site, you do need to register. Complete information is given as to what purpose registration serves and the benefits attained in doing so. Privacy is maintained through this process; however, you should carefully read the instructions for pertinent information during this process. Contact information is gathered from a feedback form available as a link on the bottom of the home page. Because this is a commercial site, the amount of advertising is not unusual; however, what is present is unobtrusive.

Upon navigating the site, you can see that the Web pages themselves are copyrighted, with individual dates. However, there seems to be no demarcation for revisions to the pages, and, in fact, unless you are looking at links that provide their own dating, it is difficult to tell the currency of links and information sites. Regardless, HealthAtoZ does a fine job of bringing together general and specific information concerning a wide array of subjects, including Basic Medical Sciences, Dental Health, Fitness, and so forth. The ease of use, brief annotations, and star rating system (defined on the About page) definitely aid users in navigating through the pages as well as in finding other relevant sites that may meet their information needs. A nice plus is that there is no distraction of frames and Java scripting, which can be highly disruptiive.

All in all, HealthAtoZ is a strong source for both consumer and professional information. The ease of use, coupled with the ability to search the entire Web site and even MEDLINE, makes it definitely one to bookmark and revisit from time to time.

Virtual Hospital
<http://www.vh.org>

Virtual Hospital is a site developed and maintained at the University of Iowa. Although certain segments of the site are for University of Iowa affiliates only (presumably because of licensing restrictions), most of the site is available to all Web users. The site contains a wealth of full-text health information as well as links to other quality sites. The mission of the Virtual Hospital is based on the philosophy that "learning is an apprenticeship, and . . . apprentice learners—health care providers and patients—need convenient access to authoritative information."[4] The site does divide its information into sources intended for providers or patients; however, it acknowledges and encourages each audience to explore all the resources of the site.

Much thought has gone into the site, intending to make it easy to use. All of the text is provided in formats that do not require helper applications, and other than the extraneous photograph-intensive home page, graphics are kept to a minimum and are not necessary for navigation. The designers have maintained a uniform style throughout the site and aim for intuitive navigation via uniform headers and footers on each page. Unfortunately, the site isn't quite as intuitive as they intend. Users new to the Web may not realize that they need to click on the text buried among the photographs on the home page to access deeper levels, and vocabulary used throughout the site, including consumer areas, assumes a fairly high comfort level with medical terminology. For example, within the For Patients section, one has the option of browsing by organ system. Although many lay users may be able to identify the major body organs, they may be overwhelmed at the next level, when they must choose among such terminology as endocrine/metabolic, hematologic, or genitourinary. Also, the choices of options are laid out in traditional lists, often necessitating lengthy scrolling through screens to find the topic wanted. Other options offered, such as word searching or browsing an annotated list, may be better suited to less educated users. Noteworthy is the inclusion of links to peer-reviewed health information sites elsewhere on the Web.

Virtual Hospital maintains a very deep commitment to authoritative information. On every page, the author is identified, as are the author's credentials, affiliation, the page's peer review status, and the revision date of the information. The electronic texts often include bibliographies, and all the text is full-text searchable so that users can find information of interest in areas of the site they might not otherwise have checked. The site often takes advantage of the strengths of the Web to deliver high-quality nontext media, such as videoclips of croup or the ankle joint. A parallel site is the Virtual Children's Hospital, laid out similar to the main Virtual Hospital site, but containing information specific to pediatrics. As with the main site, there is a wealth of full-text information as well as carefully selected links, and the user can access the information via word searching or by following the hierarchically structured links.

The Virtual Hospital contains a wealth of high-quality, authoritative information in traditional medicine. However, this authoritativeness also may make it difficult to use for less informed patients or less educated searchers. It also is largely disease centered, with minimal information on wellness beyond traditional topics such as immunization. Nevertheless, the information and links included are very high quality, and medical professionals, librarians, and more savvy patients will be very well served by this site.

PROFESSIONAL SITES

Professional megasites, unlike the other Web sites discussed in this chapter, are those which have the greatest appeal for health care professionals and academics who have specialized interests. Although consumers may find information in these sites of some interest (especially that of HealthWeb), overall, their texts and organization are most appropriate for those who have extensive knowledge in the fields of medicine and health care. The information in the sites varies greatly, but, inevitably, the terminology, types of links, and attributes are most beneficial to those who are already in the know. However, that should not discourage those who are willing and able to sift through the more technical health sciences-oriented information available on the Web.

As with the previous sections, you will find that the following sites are examples of excellent megasites, exhibiting many of the same attributes. Each has unique features that provide interesting and useful information and links to other Web sites for those needing professionally oriented resources. The following descriptions of these particular sites, similar to those previously discussed, will briefly mention quality, descriptions, production, privacy, advertising, and some unique aspects. Discussion of these attributes should be helpful in clarifying the particular Web site's role in providing resource information through the World Wide Web.

MedWeb: Biomedical Internet Resources
<http://www.medweb.emory.edu/MedWeb/>

MedWeb has been designed with both professionals and academics in mind. Organized, maintained, and revised by Emory University Health Sciences Center Library, MedWeb develops topics of special interest to health care professionals and the like. Structured by subcategories as well as alphabetically (you may choose which one to use), this site is both a megasite and a metasite. There are 8,000-plus annotated links that take you around the globe. All pages bear copyright information, and each individual page of links signifies revisions through a time date stamped on each page.

The site accepts no advertising. The question of privacy is difficult to verify, but it would be hoped that, as with many other educational institutions, only minimal information about the user is recorded for statistical reasons. As with many sites, this can only be ascertained by making inquiries directly to the Webmaster through the comments link located on each page.

What MedWeb best exemplifies, in a well-documented and balanced manner, is an organizational pattern that is consistent and quite thorough. This site, in particular, takes each topic and separates the many aspects and ways that links might be coordinated to it. For instance, the section on dermatology has categories that cover alternative medicine, guides, textbooks, and veterinary medicine. This same subject analysis is repeated for a range of subjects, such as nursing, cardiology, epidemiology, and so on. Thousands of links are made available through this method, with good results. Annotations help to identify sponsors and brief descriptions give an indication of the resources within the pages.

MedWeb is currently under reconstruction and changes should soon be evident. These changes have the potential to create a more user-friendly environment. Currently, there is a search engine available, and navigating the lists yields the best connection to links. Until the changes are complete, users will need to keep in mind that the site offers minimal explanation about its search engine and that the keywords, subcategories, and alphabetical listings will best yield the information being sought.

Cliniweb
<http://www.ohsu.edu/cliniweb/>

Cliniweb, unlike some of the sites already discussed, focuses on providing information for those who are familiar with standard indexing within the health care industry. Professionals, students in the health sciences, and practitioners will find that this site caters to their needs in a manner that puts the resources that they are likely to need in the spotlight. Produced by MNI Systems Corporation, which specializes in a variety of Internet and health care businesses, Cliniweb strives to pull together several different types of information, including an index and table of contents, MeSH (Medical Subject Heading) searching for clinical Web sites, and direct links to search MEDLINE.

The production of Cliniweb involves a diverse group of people who are identified on the About page of the Web site. Interesting enough, their professions include librarians, doctors, and nurses, each lending his or her expertise in a different way. Although there are no copyright stamps on the pages, there are revision date stamps on the browser and search results page. Because this site originates from an educational institution (Oregon Health Sciences University), there is no advertising to serve as a distraction. Privacy of the user cannot be assessed; however, since this is an educational site, one can assume that only minimal information is pulled regarding users as they access information through Cliniweb. Feedback and comments are allowed through the home page and limited on other pages.

The information obtainable through Cliniweb is highly useful to both professionals and other experienced health care workers and students. Their indexing of approximately 10,000 Web pages under the categories of anatomy and disease provide myriad links to the world. Although there is a tremendous amount of information available, Cliniweb has chosen to run a disclaimer stating the existence of "regular" search engines (such as Yahoo!, Excite, and Lycos), which have the ability to search additional sites on the Web. Still, because of its organization and subject indexing, Cliniweb is an excellent starting point for those who desire clinical information and access to medical literature on MEDLINE, offering greater precision and quality control than is provided by standard search engines.

Hardin Meta Directory
<http://www.lib.uiowa.edu/hardin/md/index.html>

The Hardin Meta Directory is a list of lists that provides access to a variety of resource sites on health-related topics. These lists include some commercial sites, such as MedWeb, Yahoo!, Martindale's Health Science Guide, Medmark, and so on. In putting this site together, Paul Soderdahl and Jim Duncan, with staff assistance from the Hardin Library for the Health Sciences (University of Iowa), have pulled together and organized a plethora of information that has mass appeal. However, it is professionals and health care-related individuals who benefit the most.

By constantly revising (and date stamping) updates to Web pages, the Hardin Meta Directory is able to provide lists that have very few dead links and that add new information on a weekly basis. Because this site provides thousands upon thousands of links, revision of pages is very important, and this site does this task very well. In addition, there is no advertising to confuse and fluster you while searching and browsing through the directory. Once again, it is difficult to assess privacy. However, one could assume that minimal information (your IP address, IP provider, etc.) is monitored as you use the site. Contact information is readily available by either directly e-mailing the Webmaster or by going to the comment page.

All in all, the Hardin Meta Directory furnishes a tremendous quantity of Web links in a neat, organized manner. Upon using the site, you will find that Hardin is easy to navigate, with its simple layering of pages, such as anesthesiology, hematology, orthopedics, and psychiatry, with additional pointers to various areas of information. By staying away from some of the fancier tools of the Internet, such as frames and Java scripting, Hardin is able to furnish easily accessible links for specific information needs.

HealthWeb
<http://healthweb.org>

HealthWeb is a Web site organized by subject areas, with consistency in the types of topics covered under each subject. Created by members of the Greater Midwest Region of the National Network of Libraries of Medicine and those of the Committee for the Institutional Cooperation of the Big Ten, it is a collaborative effort to produce a Web site that pulls together information on a number of topics of particular interest to health care professionals, academics, and students.

Each subject area is developed by one of the member libraries, with appropriate copyright and date stamps. Revisions are noted on pages as completed. Due to the educational and nonprofit status of the page, no advertising is allowed. As with many of the other pages, privacy can't truly be ascertained. For statistical purposes, it must be assumed, once again, that the Web site administrators will screen minimal information about the user. It should be noted that, although the overall site has a Webmaster, each individual subject will have a separate contact person who is specifically responsible for the information set forth on the pages.

HealthWeb's organization is highly unique. There is an extensive User Guide that gives information about databases, evaluating Internet resources, and tips on searching the Internet. Other sections include What's New, Comments, About HealthWeb, About Home-pages, and Member Libraries. Most important, the subject pages are well developed, providing information on more than eighty topics. Each topic is broken down along similar lines; for instance, the topic of nursing contains annotated lists for the following areas: Educational Resources, Listservs and Usenet Groups, Publications, and so forth. Although there are slight variations in organization, each library is held to a standard and does well in maintaining consistency throughout its respective subject areas.

With its ease of use and consistency in information available, HealthWeb makes for a pleasant Web site full of information that is readily accessible and a breeze to navigate.

Medical Matrix
<http://www.medmatrix.org/index.asp>

Medical Matrix is a peer-reviewed site providing annotated resources with numerous informative links. By concentrating on clinical information for health care professionals, this site has built an interesting niche on the World Wide Web. The authors (a full directory with links is provided) have spent an extensive amount of time pulling together the information, links, and various attributes of Medical Matrix. An editorial board, consisting of members of the American Medical Informatics Association, aids in reviewing materials and the ranking system of sites. Web surveys and comments from users are used to establish, monitor, and determine further organization of the site. There is an incredible amount of information on the background of the site, should you be interested. As with other megasites, the links on Medical Matrix are organized by subject areas. Examples are Clinical Practice, Literature, and Health-care and Professionals. A unique star system for ranking the sites, as well as feedback through the comments page to the authors, allows a higher quantity of "quality" sites available for perusal.

Revisions and new additions to the site happen on a regular basis. No advertising is present on the pages. Privacy is protected; how-ever, you must register in order to use the site. Once done, you are allowed to enter any areas of the site that you wish. Questions can be posed, and feedback offered, through the list of Web site devel-opers and/or comments page.

Medical Matrix has several unique and interesting features. Some of these include "Real Audio" Symposia (actual sound bits from symposia), Continuing Education Classes, Classifieds, and Em-ployment Opportunities. Well organized and smoothly navigable, Medical Matrix allows efficient movement through the site. The subject orientation of the site lends itself to quick and easy access, providing links to in-depth and informative sites appropriate for experienced health care professionals.

CONCLUSION

Searching for quality health care information on the Internet can be overwhelming. In addition to the anarchic, dynamic nature of the Web, the limited nature of even the best search engines makes a comprehensive, sophisticated search all but impossible. In addition, the quality of the information available on the Web ranges from excellent to downright fraudulent. Megasites, especially those in-cluded here, can help bring order to the chaos and help you find the most appropriate information. Although this chapter is far from comprehensive, it should serve as a good starting point. Depending on your situation and/or clientele, some sites will be more useful than others, but we expect that you will find among them valuable professional tools. One final caveat: the World Wide Web is a dynamic place; sites change and new, excellent examples may ap-pear. Exploring the Internet is like playing a ball game. If you hit a home run, you will want to remember how you did it and the route you took to home plate, so make sure you bookmark it!

REFERENCE NOTES

1. Newton, H. *Newton's Telecom Dictionary: The Official Dictionary of Telecommunications.* New York: Flatiron Publications, 1998.

2. Kapoun, J. "Teaching Undergrads Web Evaluation: A Guide for Library Instruction." *College & Research Libraries News* 59(July/August 1998):522-3.

3. Howe, L., Executive Editor. *WellnessWeb: Putting the HEART Back in Healthcare* [Online] (1998). Available: <http://www.wellweb.com/BIOGS.WHOAREWE.HTM>. Accessed: 18 September 1998.

4. University of Iowa. *Virtual Hospital: A Tour of the Virtual Hospital* [Online] (1998). Available: <http://www.vh.org/Welcome/VHTour.html>. Accessed: 18 September 1998.

Chapter 4

MEDLINE on the Internet

helen-ann brown
Valerie G. Rankow

INTRODUCTION

MEDLINE is the world's premier database of published biomedical journal literature, and so special attention is given in this volume to searching MEDLINE.

In this chapter, several popular MEDLINE searching systems available on the Internet are highlighted, including some free and some fee-based versions. Readers are guided through MEDLINE's scope and structure, shown how to formulate search questions for the best results, and how to evaluate search results. Several MEDLINE Internet search systems are compared using their unique and common features.

Searching each MEDLINE system using MeSH (Medical Subject Headings), the controlled vocabulary of MEDLINE, will bring better results. Only MeSH headings can be expanded or exploded, or have subheadings attached to them. Searching MEDLINE with everyday language or text words is discussed, although to properly search MEDLINE and get the best, most authoritative results, learning to use the MeSH controlled vocabulary is recommended. The complete MeSH is available online at <http://www.nlm.nih.gov/mesh/99MBrowser.html>.

Throughout the chapter, Medical Subject Headings (MeSH) are in capital letters and searching operators are shown in italics and capitalized.

What Is MEDLINE?

MEDLINE is an electronic database, created and produced by the National Library of Medicine. It is the world's foremost authority for indexing medical literature. The emphasis is on indexing journal literature of clinical medicine and medical research, as well as veterinary and dental medicine, nursing, the preclinical sciences, and health care administration.

The system you choose for searching MEDLINE on the Internet is a personal decision. Each system leads you to the same database, MEDLINE, but each may use a different way to search. Some search systems instruct you to use common everyday language to ask your search question. Some search systems are designed to use MEDLINE's controlled vocabulary, MeSH. Some search systems allow you to use a combination of everyday language and MeSH. For everyday or natural language, imagine your search system carrying your question as a train of thought, in your own words. Controlled-vocabulary searching is a structured searching language, so picture your question as sets of carefully boxed and stacked ideas.

How Is MEDLINE Organized?

The complete MEDLINE database currently includes bibliographic citations and abstracts from about 4,000 biomedical journals from all over the world, published from 1966 to the present. It is updated as frequently as every day.

When you type in your search topic, which can be an author's name, the name of a journal, significant words or phrases, MeSH headings, or any combination of these elements, the MEDLINE system manipulates your elements in the background and generates a list of literature citations that match the criteria you have selected.

The basic element of each citation is a word. A word is letters, or letters and numbers, surrounded by a space at the front and a space at the back. Words form phrases. Phrases form sentences. Sentences are phrases with a space before the first phrase and a period at the end of the last phrase, followed by at least one space. Sentences go into fields, such as the unique identifier, author field, institution field, title field, source field, subject heading field, and abstract. Fields make up the citation. The citations form the database. All MEDLINE citations contain common elements, and that is how the system can retrieve the results—the computer searches simultaneously for your criteria within these common elements.

Table 4.1 shows a sample composite citation, with the elements marked. The Unique Identifier and the PreMEDLINE ID Number are identifying numbers, similar to a Social Security number, for this article. There are four authors. MEDLINE lists up to the first ten authors of a citation. This article is written in English, as are most articles in MEDLINE. The Major MeSH Headings represent the five central topics of this article. The asterisk (*), placed in front of therapeutic use or drug therapy, means those subaspects of the MeSH headings, PULMONARY HYPERTENSION or NIFEDIPINE, are the central topic of this article. The other MeSH headings are discussed in this article, but are not the central topics. MeSH "check-tags" describe the species, gender, and ages of the subjects of the article. Registry numbers are given for the substances mentioned. The Publication Type of this article is Journal Article. This International Serials Standard Number is for the *Journal of the American College of Cardiology*. This journal is included in the A and M journal subsets. It has an abstract and is in the structured format. The address field usually has the address of the first author. This article was published in the October issue of the *Journal of the American College of Cardiology*, volume 32, issue 4, pages 1068 to 73.

MEDLINE ON THE INTERNET

At this moment, many Web sites provide access to MEDLINE. Some sites are devoted exclusively to providing MEDLINE access, or MEDLINE may be one of many databases available at a Web site. Some sites offer free access to MEDLINE, and some charge a fee. Some of the MEDLINE suppliers have designed their own searching software, whereas others link you to the National Library of Medicine's PubMed.

In fact, free and fee-based versions of MEDLINE have been available on the Internet for some time. In 1997, the National Library of Medicine (NLM) made a free version of the entire MEDLINE database available on the Internet. NLM named this searching system PubMed, perhaps because it is designed for use by the general public.

The National Library of Medicine has popularized the availability of this free system for searching the MEDLINE database, and

TABLE 4.1. A Sample Composite MEDLINE Citation. The elements are marked.

Unique Identifier	98439670
Authors	Ricciardi MJ Knight BP Martinez FJ Rubenfire M
Title	Inhaled nitric oxide in primary pulmonary hypertension: a safe and effective agent for predicting response to nifedipine.
Language	Eng
Major MeSH Heading	Calcium Channel Blockers/adverse effects/ *therapeutic use, Hypertension, Pulmonary/*drug therapy/physiopathology
	Nifedipine/adverse effects/*therapeutic use
	Nitric Oxide/*administration & dosage
	Vasodilator Agents/adverse effects/*therapeutic use
MeSH Heading	Administration, Inhalation Administration, Oral
	Hemodynamics/drug effects
	Hypotension/chemically induced
	Pulmonary Circulation/drug effects
	Vascular Resistance/drug effects
MeSH checktags	Female Human Male Middle Age
Registry Numbers of Substances	0 (Vasodilator Agents)
	10102-43-9 (Nitric Oxide)
	21829-25-4 (Nifedipine)
Publication Type	JOURNAL ARTICLE
Date of Article	19981020
Date of Publication	1998 Oct
Int'l Serial Standard Number	0735-1097
Title Abbreviation	J Am Coll Cardiol
Pages	1068-73
Subsets	A, M
Country	UNITED STATES
Issue of Publication	4
Volume of Issue	32
Journal Title Code	H50
Author Abstract	Author Entry Month - 199812
Abstract	

OBJECTIVES: The purpose of this study was to assess the utility of inhaled nitric oxide (NO), a selective pulmonary vasodilator, for predicting the safety and acute hemodynamic response to high-dose oral nifedipine in primary pulmonary hypertension (PPH). BACKGROUND: A significant decrease in pulmonary vascular resistance with an oral nifedipine challenge is predictive of an improved prognosis, and potential clinical efficacy in PPH. However, the required nifedipine trial carries significant first-dose risk of hypotension. While inhaled NO has been recommended for assessing pulmonary vasodilator reserve in PPH, it is not known whether it predicts the response to nifedipine. METHODS: Seventeen patients with PPH undergoing a nifedipine trial were assessed for hemodynamic response to inhaled NO at 80 parts per million for 5 minutes. The nifedipine trial consisted of 20 mg of nifedipine hourly for 8 hours unless limited by hypotension or intolerable side effects. Patients were classified as responders and non-responders with positive response defined as > or = 20% reduction in mean pulmonary artery pressure (mPA) or pulmonary vascular resistance (PVR) with the vasodilator administration.

RESULTS: NO was safely administered to all participants. Seven of 17 (41.2%) responded to NO, and 8 of the 17 to nifedipine (47.1%). Nifedipine was safely administered in 14 of the 17. Three suffered either mild or severe hypotension, including one death. All NO responders also responded to nifedipine, and 9 of the 10 NO nonresponders were nifedipine nonresponders, representing a sensitivity of 87.5%, specificity of 100%, and overall predictive accuracy of 94%. All NO responders tolerated a full nifedipine trial without hypotension. There was a highly significant correlation between the effects of NO and nifedipine on PVR (r=0.67, p=0.003).
CONCLUSIONS: The pulmonary vascular response to inhaled NO accurately predicts the acute hemodynamic response to nifedipine in PPH, and a positive response to NO is associated with a safe nifedipine trial. In patients comparable with those evaluated, a trial of nifedipine in NO nonresponders appears unwarranted and potentially dangerous.

Address	Department of Internal Medicine, University of Michigan, Ann Arbor, USA.
PreMEDLINE ID number	0009768734
Source	J Am Coll Cardiol 1998 Oct;32(4):1068-73

consumers and health care professionals are responding. Over 12 million people had searched PubMed each month, as of November 1998, according to a National Library of Medicine spokesperson. In June 1997, 18,000 people had used PubMed. By December 1997, the number had almost doubled, to 34,000 daily users. By November 1998, the number of PubMed users had more than doubled again, with over 70,000 users of PubMed per day.

However, even with PubMed available, searchers still chose other Web sites that maintain a link to MEDLINE, both free and fee-based, because they prefer the extra features of these other searching systems, or just out of familiarity—the comfort factor.

Whether for a fee or for free, some things are the same in all the Internet versions of MEDLINE examined, but there are enough subtle and not so subtle differences that your search results can be completely skewed if you are not using the system correctly. For example, most of the searching systems allow the use of positional operators *ADJACENCY (ADJ)*, *WITH*, or *NEAR*. Also, most of the searching systems allow the use of the Boolean operators *AND* and *OR*. Either *AND* or *OR* may be designated the default operator. The default operator is the one the system will automatically use if you do not specify a search operator. It is strongly recommended that you read the help files before you begin to search.

Each system lets you browse through MEDLINE's citations. The full MEDLINE database, from 1966 to the present, contains almost

11 million citations, most now with abstracts. Differences between the systems include how many years are covered, whether the vendor offers a link to the full text of an article, or whether there is a simple and convenient way to order the full text of the articles. Some systems will offer you a link to the publisher's Web site, where you can find the full text of an article or a way to order the full text of the articles.

Table 4.2 is a list of the free and fee-based systems that will be discussed, with their Internet addresses. A comparison of the similarities and differences between these MEDLINE search systems will be made later in this chapter.

TABLE 4.2. List of MEDLINE Searching Systems and Internet Addresses

MEDLINE Searching System	Internet Address
Free	
Avicenna	http://www.avicenna.com
BioMedNet	http://biomednet.com
HealthGate	http://www.healthgate.com
Infotrieve	http://www.infotrieve.com
Medscape	http://www.medscape.com
PubMed	http://www.nlm.nih.gov
Fee Based	
Aries Knowledge Finder	http://www.kfinder.com
DIALOG	http://www.dialogweb.com
OCLC FirstSearch	http://www.oclc.org/oclc/fs/logon.htm
Ovid Technologies	http://gateway.ovid.com

SEARCHING MEDLINE

How do you formulate your MEDLINE search question? First, what do you want to know? Formulating your search question is the most important step in planning to search MEDLINE. Once you decide on your question, you carefully follow the directions of the MEDLINE searching system you have selected.

Be specific. Plan to search for tennis elbow, instead of sports injuries. Plan to search for Adriamycin, instead of antineoplastic agents. If your search topic focuses on particular persons, particular tests or procedures, any comparisons, or any outcomes, include them in your strategy.

The elements of a MEDLINE citation include author, title, journal name, an institution, publication date, and subject headings or descriptors (see Table 4.1). You may look for any one element or some combination. You may already know some of the elements, such as the author and publication date, or just have an idea of a subject. You may know the specific treatment, drug name, or procedure, and you may have a specific diagnosis or condition. If you have that information, your search topic should be specific.

Once you formulate a specific topic, also consider what you plan to do with the information you find. If you need to make a patient care decision, find a drug or treatment for a particular disease, or make a brief presentation, you will require less literature than if you have to give a conference presentation or write a review paper or a grant proposal.

What type of literature do you want? MEDLINE contains literature in different publication types, including case reports, editorials, letters, reviews, meta-analyses, clinical trials, and randomized controlled trials. Do you want only very recent literature, or do you want to search over a longer period of time? MEDLINE covers journal literature from 1966 to the present.

Important questions to answer as you formulate your search are presented in Table 4.3. In your searching process, you will formulate your search question and represent each concept with words, phrases, MeSH headings, or a combination of search elements. Next,

TABLE 4.3. Important Questions to Answer As You Formulate Your Search

1. What topic do you want to search?
   a. Any particular age group, gender, or ethnic group?
   b. Are you concerned about cause of disease, method of diagnosis, ways to treat, or prognosis?
2. What will you do with this information, and, therefore, how much information do you need?
3. How many years of publication are you looking for?
4. What kind of publication are you looking for?
   a. An overview article is a REVIEW, TUTORIAL.
   b. For drug therapy studies, RANDOMIZED CONTROLLED TRIAL is preferred.
5. Do you expect to find a large or small amount of information?

you decide which search operator or search operators will put your concepts together. If you have used natural search language with words and/or phrases, choose positional or proximity operators. If you have used authors' names, journal titles, the name of an institution, or MeSH headings, use Boolean operators to join your search elements together.

The Boolean operator *AND* will join all your concepts together, for example, HEADACHE *AND* ASPIRIN *AND* Innsbruck (institution) *AND* Burtscher M (author). The Boolean operator *OR* will group concepts or synonyms together, for example, aspirin or Tylenol or ibuprofen or Advil or acetaminophen. You will retrieve citations on each drug alone or citations that discuss more than one drug.

The positional operators *ADJACENCY, WITH,* or *NEAR* will bring your words together, in phrases in exact order, within so many words, or words near each other. The *ADJACENCY* operator retrieves words in phrases in exact order, with no other words in between. The first word is followed by the second, which is followed by the third. Chinese *ADJ* Restaurant *ADJ* Syndrome retrieves citations about Chinese Restaurant Syndrome. This is the allergic reaction to MSG (monosodium glutamate) used in preparing Chinese dishes.

In some systems, such as Ovid, *ADJACENCY* is the default positional operator. The Ovid system will automatically place the *ADJACENCY* operator in between the words and then perform the search. The searcher types in, world wide web. Ovid translates the phrase to world *ADJ* wide *ADJ* web and then performs the search.

The *WITH* operator spreads the words in phrases apart and usually allows for a different word order. You can designate within how many words your significant words need to appear in citation titles, MeSH headings, and abstracts. For example, you are looking for the use of time-released cough remedies. You enter the search statement time *W5* released *W5* cough *W5* remedies. Any arrangement of these words within five words of each other will be relevant for you. You retrieve a citation titled "Cough Remedies Now Come in Time-Released Formulas." You retrieve another citation titled "Remedies for Your Cough Are Released Over Time." Within an abstract, you may find a sentence such as "Johnson and Johnson introduces a line of time-released cough remedies for children and adults." Within another abstract, you may find a sentence such as, "Cough remedies released over time allow children to sleep through the night."

There is no *WITH* operator in Ovid. A number used with the *ADJACENCY* operator, such as *ADJ5*, operates the same as the *WITH* operator. In OCLC FirstSearch, the *WITH* operator spreads the words apart, but they must remain in the same order. If you were looking for allergies to various types of chocolate, you could enter allergies *W3* chocolate in OCLC FirstSearch. You would retrieve the phrases allergies to milk chocolate, allergies to dark chocolate, or allergies to semisweet chocolate with that strategy.

The *NEAR* operator retrieves words in phrases near each other, in any order. This encompasses words in exact order, in reversed order, within so many words, and words nearby. For example, you are looking for citations that discuss motorized vans to carry wheelchairs. Your search strategy, motorized *N5* vans *N5* wheelchairs, will retrieve titles such as "Vans Come Motorized to Lift and Then Carry Wheelchairs" or "Wheelchairs Demand Vans to Come Motorized with Rear Wheel Lifts."

The Boolean operators *AND* and *OR* are used when handling authors, journal titles, and MeSH headings. The positional operators *ADJACENCY, WITH,* and *NEAR* are used when handling significant words in phrases in citation titles and abstracts. It is possible that you will use both types of searching operators in one search. For example:

> *Search topic:* Evaluation of patient education or consumer health information available on the Internet.

> 1. PATIENT EDUCATION *OR* (consumer *W3* health *W3* information)
> 2. Internet *OR* World *ADJ* Wide *ADJ* Web
> 3. 1 *AND* 2

How Do You Enter Your Search Topic?

Most MEDLINE systems offer a basic and advanced mode of searching. On a basic search screen, the system will ask you to write your search topic using natural or everyday language. You can easily type in the search topic "harm to children from front seat airbags." Behind the scenes, the MEDLINE system is translating your search into words, phrases, MeSH headings, or a combination of these search elements and then joining the concepts together with Boolean and positional operators.

When the system searched for the phrase "front seat airbags," it would have found the MeSH heading AIRBAG. It may have used the word "harm" or chosen to attach the subheading adverse effects or contraindications to the MeSH heading AIRBAG. It used the MeSH checktag CHILD. The MEDLINE system used the Boolean searching operator *AND* to join the search concepts together.

Many Web-based MEDLINE systems also have an advanced mode. You will need to have some knowledge of MEDLINE searching mechanics, such as how to enter an author's name, how to enter a journal title, how and when to use MeSH headings or text words, using searching operators, and using truncation to retrieve a variety of middle letters or endings of a particular word.

By using a truncation symbol, such as a ":" or a "#" or a "?" at the end of a text word root or trunk, you are instructing the MEDLINE searching system to include any version of the word in the search strategy. It is a shortcut to *OR*ing the noun, adjective, adverb, gerund, or participle variants of a text word. The root treat: will retrieve treat, treats, treated, treating, and treatment. Extend the word root or trunk as far as you can before placing the truncation symbol. However, sometimes you will get text words you do not want. You want rat or rats, but by entering rat#, you will also get rata or rate. You want arm or arms, but by entering arm?, you will also get armadillo.

In some MEDLINE systems, you can display a list of available forms of the word and then select the ones you want. In other MEDLINE systems, you can designate up to how many extra letters you want added to the end of the word. Also, in some MEDLINE systems, you can place a truncation symbol within a word to get variations. Tum?r will bring the British spelling of tumour as well as the American spelling, tumor. Aries Knowledge Finder automatically searches every word variant, unless you turn off that feature.

An advanced mode lets you enter your search step by step. The MEDLINE system will probably have several lines to fill in where you can select the field names. Use the Help screen to assist you.

Using the same search topic, harm to children from front seat airbags, the MeSH heading AIRBAG with the subheading AE (adverse effects), AIRBAG/AE, is displayed. The word "front" and the MeSH checktag CHILD are displayed. Choose the *AND* operator to join your three ideas together.

MeSH headings, such as ACCIDENTS or HYPERTENSION, can be exploded or expanded to include both broad and narrow related search terms. For example, the MeSH term HYPERTENSION can be exploded to include all the narrower terms relating to that subject:

HYPERTENSION, MALIGNANT
HYPERTENSION, PORTAL
HYPERTENSION, PULMONARY
HYPERTENSION, RENAL

However, in most MEDLINE systems, the MeSH heading does not include the narrower terms unless the searcher explodes the term and the MEDLINE system *OR*s the broader term with the narrower related search terms. Most MEDLINE systems do not automatically explode. The searcher must select that feature. Notable exceptions are PubMed and Aries Knowledge Finder.

Many MEDLINE systems will display a list of citations ranked by most relevant first. Each system applies an elaborate searching algorithm to the citation list to determine which citation is the best match. Your words probably have appeared in the citation title, major MeSH position, and many times in the abstract to be in first position. Some MEDLINE systems display the citations by most recent first. The last citations added to the database are the first ones you see.

Many MEDLINE systems now link to the full text of an article by linking to the journal's Web page. Some MEDLINE systems have the full text of certain journals available as a database to which you can subscribe. Almost all the MEDLINE systems can lead you to a document delivery system to mail, fax, or electronically send you a copy of your article for a fee, or you can contact and do business with any document delivery provider.

Table 4.4 is a comparative chart of some popular MEDLINE searching systems. Cost, years of coverage, availability of MeSH,

TABLE 4.4. Comparative Chart of MEDLINE Searching Systems

MEDLINE System Delivery? URL	Fee?	Years?	Built-in MeSH?	Link Document to Full Text?
Avicenna yes http://www.avicenna.com	no register	1990-	separate MeSH	no
BioMedNet no http://biomednet.com	no	1966-	yes	yes
HealthGate yes http://www.healthgate.com	no	last 2 years	ReADER maps to MeSH	yes
Infotrieve yes http://www.infotrieve.com	no register	1966- several files	yes	yes
Medscape yes http://www.medscape.com	no register	1985-	yes	yes
PubMed yes http://nlm.nih.gov	no	1966- one file	MeSH browser	yes
Aries Knowledge Finder no http://www.kfinder.com	yes	1966-	no	no
Dialog Web yes http://www.dialogweb.com	yes	1966-	separate database	yes
OCLC FirstSearch yes http://www.oclc.org/pclc/fs/ logon.htm	yes	1966-	can browse related subjects, keywords	yes
Ovid no http://gateway.ovid.com	yes	1966-	yes	4 full-text databases

links to full text, and availability of document delivery were criteria for comparison.

SELECTED WEB-BASED MEDLINE SYSTEMS

The MEDLINE searching systems listed in Table 4.4 were scrutinized using a search strategy combining the drug NIFEDIPINE and the condition HYPERTENSION. The different versions of MEDLINE share some common features, but also have some very strong differences. Again, you should read the help file for each system to learn the best way to formulate your search and to help guarantee that you will retrieve the results you want.

Avicenna, BioMedNet, HealthGate, Infotrieve, Medscape, and PubMed are free. You must register to use Avicenna, Infotrieve, and Medscape. Aries Knowledge Finder, DIALOG, OCLC FirstSearch, and Ovid are fee based; prices vary from fees per printed citation to fees based on the number of users accessing the system simultaneously.

Most of these systems search MEDLINE from 1966 to the present. Aries Knowledge Finder, BioMedNet, DIALOG, and PubMed search from 1966 to the present in one file. Ovid and Infotrieve cover all the years, although not necessarily in one pass. Avicenna covers from 1990 to the present. HealthGate searches the last two years in basic mode.

All of these systems offer an option for Boolean searching. You can *AND* or *OR* your searching concepts. Some systems also offer a variety of positional operators, such as *ADJ*, *WITH*, or *NEAR*.

All of these MEDLINE searching systems offer a basic and advanced mode for entering your search concepts. The basic mode is recommended for less experienced searchers and those who will search less often. The advanced mode is for more experienced users.

These MEDLINE systems display available citations and offer a way to link to the full text of the citation or arrange for you to receive the full text through a document delivery system. Most will display the citations ranked by best match first, or relevancy. Ovid displays results by most recent date first. All systems offer Help screens or tips to searching. Use them to ensure accuracy.

Searching MEDLINE on the Internet is a dynamic experience. Change is the only certainty. The following paragraphs highlight unique features of these selected MEDLINE searching systems, as of January 1999.

Free MEDLINE Systems

Avicenna
<www.avicenna.com>

Avicenna applies a fuzzy Boolean logic searching strategy. Fuzzy logic will rank the citations by best match first. Boolean logic will *AND* and *OR* your searching terms. Avicenna only has one Help file for both basic and advanced methods of searching, even though there are separate screens for the basic and advanced searching modes. On the basic screen there are two choices for finding citations with your significant words. "All words found, unranked" will *AND* your words; every citation will contain each of your words. "Any words found, ranked" will *OR* your words; every citation will have at least one of your words.

You can select automatic plurals and have the system search the words "scan" and "scans" at the same time. It will not, however, search "tooth" and "teeth" for you at the same time. Avicenna does not map to MeSH. It does not translate the phrase "high blood pressure" to the MeSH heading HYPERTENSION. However, the Avicenna system offers a separate MeSH file for you to look up the correct MeSH heading to use for the phrase "high blood pressure."

The advanced searching page has a box for you to enter words to be found in the titles of your documents. Here, you could create ideal citation titles. There is also a box for searching a personal name as a subject. This feature will retrieve citations about Abraham Lincoln or Arthur Ashe, for example.

BioMedNet
<www.biomednet.com>

BioMedNet's "Evaluated MEDLINE" offers easy to understand Help screens. The name Evaluated MEDLINE comes from the evaluation of some MEDLINE citations as outstanding. These are citations from articles published in full-text journals that are available through BioMedNet and cited in the series of Current Opinion journals, such as *Current Opinion in Oncology.* In the MEDLINE + citations format, you will see either "e*" or "e**" within a citation to indicate an "evaluated" citation.

BioMedNet has the same related-articles feature as PubMed, courtesy of the PubMed searching system. There is extensive linking to full-text articles, but you will be charged for each copy of a full-text article.

BioMedNet's MEDLINE searching system remembers your search history during your current search session and for future sessions. You can combine search statement #1 and search statement #2 during this session. When you log in a week later, your search strategy is still displayed.

The stemming feature is the truncation feature. To explode a MeSH heading, you must select a term from the MeSH Tree display and then click on it with the magnifying glass.

HealthGate
<www.healthgate.com>

HealthGate offers clear and concise Help screens. A subheading can be attached to a natural language phrase. To search for the therapy of high blood pressure, you can enter "high-blood-pressure-th." Or, to search for therapy of lung cancer, you may enter "lung-cancer-th." The words and the two-letter subheading abbreviation must be bound by hyphens.

ReADER software maps concept words to MeSH headings. In the basic search, the ReADER feature is on and cannot be turned off. *AND* is the searching operator in the basic search mode. All of your concepts will be joined together and each will appear in the list of citations.

The advanced searching mode offers *AND*, *OR*, *NOT*, and *ADJACENCY* as search operators. This searching mode also includes more years of coverage and other searching limits. Using ReADER, you can turn off the MeSH mapping feature. When it is on, your searching concepts will be *AND*ed. When ReADER is off, you can apply the other searching operators, such as *OR, NOT,* or *AD-JACENCY.*

As with Avicenna, HealthGate has the automatic plurals feature. This system displays your search query in an attractive easy-to-follow manner.

Infotrieve
<www.infotrieve.com>

You can search from 1966 to the present in Infotrieve; however, you need to check several blocks of years, instead of only one box. Your search words are highlighted in bold and italics, so you can easily spot them in the citation titles, abstracts, and list of MeSH headings.

There is only one searching screen. The top box is similar to other basic search screens, and the other boxes resemble the system screens for advanced searching. Infotrieve encourages searchers to enter a search statement in "natural conversational syntax" in the top searching box. Phrases are entered surrounded by single quotes, 'high blood pressure,' or with the *ADJACENCY* operator between the words, for example, high *ADJ* blood *ADJ* pressure.

Infotrieve displays many searching features in an elaborate chart. The chart includes the asterisk (*) as the truncation symbol for any string of characters. You can enter micro* to retrieve the words microwave, microtubules, or microvascular. You can enter *icillin to retrieve the words ampicillin, penicillin, or amoxicillin.

Medscape
<www.medscape.com>

Medscape, similar to PubMed, displays Help in a separate window. You can have your searching screen and Help screen open at the same time. *OR* is the searching default. Any and all of your search concepts will be searched.

Besides the Boolean operators *AND, OR, NOT,* you can apply the *WITH* operator and even designate the number of words within which to find your search concepts. You can enter *W/8* to designate finding your search concepts within eight words of each other. The search statement "portable *W8* home *W8* dialysis" retrieves citations with titles or phrases in the abstracts such as "Portable dialysis allows patients to receive treatment at home," or "Dialysis is possible at home with a portable machine."

As with Infotrieve, field labels can be displayed at the end of a searching concept following a colon (:). For articles written by John Glenn, you would enter Glenn J: AU. A phrase nested in parentheses with the ":MH" qualifier for MeSH heading will map to the proper MeSH heading. If you enter, "(high blood pressure):MH," Medscape maps to the MeSH heading HYPERTENSION.

Medscape has a weekly current awareness service called Med-Pulse. It is delivered by electronic mail. You set up a profile of health-related topics important to you, and each week your customized message features new Medscape entries on those topics. Many of these items will be full-text documents compiled by Medscape staff.

PubMed
<www.nlm.nih.gov>

PubMed automatically explodes MeSH headings and searches from 1966 to the present. In the basic searching mode, words are mapped to MeSH headings and also searched as words. "High blood pressure" would be searched as words, and the MeSH heading HYPERTENSION would be *OR*ed with that retrieval.

The Help screen is separate from the search screen and can be kept open while you search. The PubMed Help system is thorough and detailed, and using it makes searching PubMed much easier. The Help screen demonstrates many features not mentioned on the same page as the search screens.

Words enclosed in quotation marks will be considered a phrase and searched as words next to each other. "High blood pressure" will be searched as the phrase, not the individual words, high, blood, and pressure. In the basic mode you can enter Boolean operators in your strategy. *AND*, *OR*, and *NOT* must be capitalized to be recognized as Boolean operators.

The "details" button will show you the search strategy PubMed created and searched for you. You may also enter field label qualifiers to distinguish authors names or journal title abbreviations.

These are entered surrounded by square brackets, "[ ]". If you wanted to find articles published in the *New England Journal of Medicine*, you would enter N Engl J Med[ta] into PubMed.

In the advanced searching mode, you can have the system process your search automatically or have it list available MeSH or text words for you, and then you make the selection. You may even start your search in the MeSH Browser by looking for ways to represent your searching concepts. As you choose them, they are placed into your searching strategy.

PubMed has developed the "related articles" feature. When you find a quality citation, you can click on related articles, and PubMed will find other articles for you very similar to that one. BioMedNet uses this feature, borrowed from PubMed. Also, since PubMed uses Entrez searching software from the National Center for Biotechnology Information, it offers links to viewing gene structures and protein structures for substances mentioned in your citation list.

Fee-Based MEDLINE Systems

The fee-based systems, such as Aries Knowledge Finder, DIALOG, OCLC FirstSearch, and Ovid, offer you a subscription to access a family of databases, including MEDLINE. Each has its own software system. The database providers hope the searcher will find their software so powerful or feature rich, that the searcher will choose fee-based over free systems. The software features that make one MEDLINE searching system more desirable than another are based on personal preferences, whether free or fee based.

Aries Knowledge Finder
<www.kfinder.com>

Aries Knowledge Finder was the first system to introduce fuzzy logic searching. As with so many MEDLINE searching systems created after it, you type one or two significant words in the search box, and the system generates a list of citations ranked best match first. When using fuzzy logic, you can now choose to have your concepts mapped to words, concepts, and synonyms. For example, CABG will be mapped to coronary artery bypass grafting.

Boolean searching is also available, with *AND* as the default operator. If you want to use *OR*, you need to type it in. Knowledge Finder also automatically explodes MeSH headings, and it will search all spelling variations of a word. If you search with the word "manage," the system will *OR* the words managing, management, and managed. All of these personalized searching features are set in a pop-up search control box. After a brief free demonstration period, there is a fee to search Knowledge Finder.

DIALOG
<www.dialogweb.com>

DIALOG places MEDLINE in its medicine category, with other similar databases such as EMBASE and BIOSIS. A preview search of this category can be performed in DialIndex, and you can see if MEDLINE is the best database for your health-related question. If you decide to run your search only in MEDLINE, you can perform a guided search, targeted search, or command language search. The guided search is closest to a basic search. The targeted search represents frequently asked search questions. If you search more than one database, DIALOG offers a Remove Duplicates feature. LIMITALL allows you to apply limits to an entire search session. You fill in ready-made search forms and retrieve citations to specific questions, for example, finding papers by a particular author.

In command search mode, you need to know DIALOG searching language. However, Help files, called Blue Sheets, are linked to your MEDLINE searching screen. Your search strategy can be saved for another session or converted to a strategy for an "Alert" automatic update. DIALOG displays the results on a "picklist page." It shows the cost of a full record.

OCLC FirstSearch
<www.oclc.org/oclc/fs/logon.htm>

MEDLINE is in the medicine and health science family of databases. The basic search box *AND*s the words you type in. A list of titles is displayed. You tag the record, show the record, and then print or e-mail the selected records. Also, FirstSearch links to the

OCLC holdings databases and shows a table of which library holds the journals cited in your records. From that point, you can command the system to get your item. If you want to add another aspect to your search, you can display the history of your basic search and narrow your retrieval by *AND*ing additional terms. You can also narrow your retrieval by selecting up to three additional subjects from a list of MeSH suggestions. You can perform a more elaborate search on the advanced searching screen. Limits to year, publication type, and language are available. On each screen, you can choose in which field you want your words searched. Default will search the most common fields, such as author, title, abstract, or MeSH.

At every step of your search, easy-to-understand help is offered. Tables show searching features and what each "tells FirstSearch" to do. Institutions subscribe to FirstSearch and purchase blocks of searching time for their patrons.

Ovid
<http://gateway.Ovid.com>

Ovid offers many features. You can turn on a map to the MeSH heading feature, and Ovid will display applicable MeSH headings. For the concept of high blood pressure, Ovid will display the MeSH headings HYPERTENSION, BLOOD PRESSURE, ANTIHYPER-TENSIVE AGENTS and the word phrase "high blood pressure." When you choose one heading, it will then display the heading's tree structure.

The tree structures display the broader and more specific headings surrounding a MeSH heading. You must decide if you want the term you typed in *OR*ed, with each of the more specific MeSH headings indented under it.

If you want any one of those MeSH headings or any combination of those MeSH headings, explode the MeSH heading. If you want the entire category, or more than one specific term within the category, explode. Ovid has added one option for automatic exploding. This is a system change option.

If you want only one specific term, you should choose that term, and only that term. If you want one, or two, or a select number of MeSH headings from the tree structure display, check off only those boxes and do not choose to explode. The next screen displays allowable subheadings, from which you would select appropriate concepts.

There are also limits for age, language, and publication types. For questions using NIFEDIPINE for HYPERTENSION, if you select RANDOMIZED CONTROLLED TRIAL as your publication type, it means the articles will all involve clinical trials using randomly selected subjects. If available, the limit to Best Evidence will filter your MEDLINE retrieval to high-quality citations. The following section discusses using the advanced Evidence-Based Medicine search concepts.

As with the other fee-based MEDLINE systems mentioned, Ovid can be part of a local intranet. MEDLINE in your Ovid system can be linked to several additional databases in the Ovid collection of databases. The Core Biomedical Collections offer full text of the MEDLINE citations.

HOW DO YOU EVALUATE YOUR RESULTS?
(EVIDENCE-BASED MEDICINE)

Note: This section is for advanced searchers; others should skip to the chapter summary on p. 75.

Your goal is to retrieve high-quality citations. A high-quality citation will describe solid study methodology and base its conclusions on the results obtained from this solid study methodology. You are looking for prospective studies with a large sample of patients that have been randomized, blinded, and controlled. You are looking for studies that have reached statistically significant results.

These concepts are part of Evidence-Based Medicine or Evidence-Based Practice. You can pose the questions "Would someone base their medical practice on the evidence presented in the study at this time?"; "Are the results of the study valid?"; and "How do these results help me in my practice?" to help you to determine the quality of the study.

To determine if you retrieved quality citations, you can examine the titles, MeSH headings, and publication types of the records you have retrieved and look for certain items, or you can incorporate MeSH headings and publication types in your search strategy to be sure these terms will be in your retrieved citations. If you are examining your retrieved titles, watch for words such as randomized, controlled, prospective, or double-blind. If you are reviewing MeSH headings, watch for terms such as PROSPECTIVE STUDY, DOUBLE-BLIND METHOD, SENSITIVITY AND SPECIFICITY, REPRODUCIBILITY OF RESULTS, and PREDICTIVE VALUE OF TESTS. If you are reviewing publication types, watch for RANDOMIZED CONTROLLED TRIAL, CLINICAL TRIAL, and MULTICENTER STUDY.

It is preferable to incorporate Evidence-Based Medicine searching techniques in your initial search strategy. You will retrieve fewer, better articles to review. There are four main Evidence-Based Medicine searching techniques: therapy, diagnosis, etiology or harm, and prognosis. Following are some simple things you can do to start searching with Evidence-Based Medicine techniques.

Therapy

To retrieve quality articles on different types of therapy, including drug therapy, attach the THERAPEUTIC USE subheading to the substance and attach the subheading THERAPY or PREVENTION AND CONTROL or DRUG THERAPY to the disease. *AND* the two concepts together. Limit the results for language, human, and/or a particular age group. Also, limit for RANDOMIZED CONTROLLED TRIAL.

An example would be if you needed to find high-quality articles on the use of Naprosyn for rheumatoid arthritis. Your first search statement could be NAPROSYN/TU. Your second search statement could be ARTHRITIS, RHEUMATOID/DT,PC,TH. Your third search statement could be 1 *AND* 2. Your fourth search statement would begin the limits, with limiting to RANDOMIZED CONTROLLED TRIAL. Finally, you could limit to English language and HUMAN. Table 4.5 displays this sample search strategy, along with a sample citation.

Diagnosis

The Evidence-Based Medicine searching techniques to retrieve quality citations on diagnostic technique include using the subhead-

TABLE 4.5. Example of Search Strategy Formulation to Retrieve Citations on Quality Therapy

---

Search question: Is naprosyn used to treat rheumatoid arthritis?

1. NAPROSYN/TU
2. ARTHRITIS, RHEUMATOID/DT,PC,TH
3. 1 *AND* 2
4. Limit to RANDOMIZED CONTROLLED TRIAL
5. Limit to English and Human

Authors	Lisse JR.
Institution	Division of Rheumatology, University of Texas Medical Branch, Galveston, USA.
Title	Clinical efficacy and safety of Naprelan versus Naprosyn in the treatment of rheumatoid arthritis.
Source	American Journal of Orthopedics. 25(9 Suppl):21-9, 1996 Sep.
Major MeSH headings:	*Anti-Inflammatory Agents, Non-Steroidal / tu [Therapeutic Use] *Arthritis, Rheumatoid / dt [Drug Therapy] *Naproxen / tu [Therapeutic Use]
MeSH Headings	Anti-Inflammatory Agents, Non-Steroidal / ad [Administration & Dosage] Anti-Inflammatory Agents, Non-Steroidal / ae [Adverse Effects] Comparative Study Delayed-Action Preparations Double-Blind Method Drug Administration Schedule Gastrointestinal Diseases / ci [Chemically Induced] Naproxen / ad [Administration & Dosage] Naproxen / ae [Adverse Effects] Safety
MeSH checktags	Adult, Aged, Female, Human, Male, Middle Age
Registry Numbers	0 (Anti-Inflammatory Agents, Non-Steroidal). 0 (Delayed-Action Preparations). 22204-53-1 (Naproxen).
Publication Type	Randomized Controlled Trial
Abstract	

A double-blind, randomized study compared the efficacy and safety of a controlled-release naproxen sodium formulation (Naprelan, Wyeth-Ayerst Laboratories, Philadelphia, Pennsylvania) 1,000 mg once daily; a conventional naproxen formulation (Naprosyn, Syntex Laboratories, Inc., Palo Alto, California) 500 mg BID; and placebo given for 12 weeks to 348 patients with rheumatoid arthritis (RA). This was followed by an open-label study to evaluate the safety of naprelan 1,000 mg once daily for an additional 9 months. In the double-blind phase of this study, the safety and efficacy of Naprelan 1,000 mg once daily were compared with those of Naprosyn 500 mg twice daily and placebo in 348 patients with RA. At the end of 12 weeks of treatment, Naprelan and Naprosyn were numerically superior to placebo in 3 of the 4 primary efficacy variables—physician's global assessment, patient's global assessment, and number of painful joints. Differences between Naprelan and placebo reached statistical significance for the patient's global assessment at Week 12 (Visit 7). Significantly more Naprosyn- than placebo-treated patients had at least 1 severe digestive system adverse event (AE); 1 drug-related AE; or 1 drug-related, digestive-system AE. There was no statistically significant difference in the number of AEs experienced by Naprelan-treated patients compared

TABLE 4.5 *(continued)*

with those who received placebo. A total of 240 patients enrolled in the Naprelan open-label phase. As would be expected, patients initially treated with placebo showed significant improvement after starting Naprelan. Those initially receiving Naprelan or Naprosyn also maintained their improvement. The AE profile with Naprelan was similar to that reported in the double-blind phase. It was concluded that Naprelan 1,000 mg once daily was as effective as Naprosyn 500 mg BID in the treatment of RA and was particularly effective in relieving pain later in the day. The controlled-release formulation may also offer safety benefits.

ings DIAGNOSIS, DIAGNOSTIC USE, and the explosion of the MeSH heading SENSITIVITY AND SPECIFICITY.

For example, use evidence-based searching techniques if you need to find quality articles on whether the purified protein derivative (PPD) test is still reliable in diagnosing pulmonary tuberculosis. You can use PPD as a text word appearing in the title or abstract or MeSH heading. However, remember you can only attach subheadings to MeSH headings. Using the MeSH heading, TUBERCULIN TEST you can attach the subheading DIAGNOSTIC USE: TUBERCULIN TEST/DU. If you took the text word and MeSH heading approach, *OR* those results to have one search statement of diagnostic use.

In the next search statement, you can enter TUBERCULOSIS, PULMONARY/DI. Join the two concepts, the tests, and the diagnosis of the disease. In the next search statement, apply the quality filter by *AND*ing in the explosion of SENSITIVITY AND SPECIFICITY. The explosion brings you citations on SENSITIVITY AND SPECIFICITY, PREDICTIVE VALUE OF TESTS, and the ROC CURVE. This search strategy is displayed in Table 4.6, followed by a sample citation.

Cause or Harm

The Evidence-Based Medicine searching techniques to retrieve quality citations on cause or harm include the use of the subheadings ETIOLOGY, CHEMICALLY INDUCED, ADVERSE EFFECTS, POISONING, TOXICITY, and EPIDEMIOLOGY, as well

TABLE 4.6. Example of Search Strategy Formulation to Retrieve Citations on Quality Diagnosis

Search question: Is the PPD test still reliable in diagnosing pulmonary tuberculosis?

1. ppd
2. TUBERCULIN TEST/DU
3. 1 *OR* 2
4. PULMONARY TUBERCULOSIS/DI
5. 3 *AND* 4
6. 5 *AND* EXP SENSITIVITY AND SPECIFICITY
7. Limit to English and Human

Authors	Huebner RE, Schein MF, Cauthen GM, Geiter LJ, Selin MJ, Good RC, O'Brien RJ.
Institution	Division of Tuberculosis Elimination, Centers for Disease Control, Atlanta, Georgia 30333.
Title	Evaluation of the clinical usefulness of mycobacterial skin test antigens in adults with pulmonary mycobacterioses.
Source	American Review of Respiratory Disease. 145(5):1160-6, 1992 May.
Major MeSH Headings	Mycobacterium avium-intracellulare Infection / di [Diagnosis] *Mycobacterium Infections, Atypical / di [Diagnosis] *Tuberculin / im [Immunology] *Tuberculin Test *Tuberculosis, Pulmonary / di [Diagnosis]
MeSH Headings	Comparative Study Double-Blind Method Evaluation Studies Micobacterium avium Complex / im [Immunology] Mycobacterium bovis / im [Immunology] Predictive Value of Tests Sensitivity and Specificity
MeSH checktags	Female, Human, Male, Middle Age
Publication Type	Clinical Trial. Controlled Clinical Trial. Journal Article. Multicenter Study.

Abstract

A double-blind, multicenter study was conducted to evaluate the usefulness of mycobacterial skin test antigens for the specific diagnosis of adult pulmonary mycobacterial disease. The skin test antigens used were PPD-T (M. bovis) and PPD-B (M. intracellular), made bioequivalent to 5 TU PPD-S through bioassay in human subjects. Of the 192 adults (18 yr of age or older), those with disease caused by M. tuberculosis (MTB) had significantly larger reactions to PPD-T than did those with disease caused by nontuberculous mycobacteria (NTM) or those with negative culture results (NEG)(13.41 mm versus 4.87 and 4.96 mm, respectively, p less than 0.001). The mean induration to PPD-B in NTM was not different from that in MTB or NEG. Defining a "positive" to be greater than or equal to 10 mm induration and a size difference of greater than or equal to 3 mm between PPD-T and PPD-B, the sensitivity, specificity, and positive predictive value (PPV) for PPD-T in diagnosing MTB versus NTM was 29, 90, and 75%. Corresponding values for PPD-B and NTM disease were 70, 61, and 64%. Dual testing was less useful in distinguishing disease caused by any of the mycobacteria from NEG. Although the sensitivity of PPD-B, made bioequivalent to PPD-S, was high, the specificity and PPV were low. We conclude that this preparation of PPD-B is no more useful in distinguishing adult pulmonary disease caused by NTM than is PPD-T alone.

as the explosion of the MeSH heading EPIDEMIOLOGIC STUDY CHARACTERISTICS. This explosion will include the MeSH headings COHORT STUDIES, PROSPECTIVE STUDIES, and LONGITUDINAL STUDIES.

In this sample search, you need to find citations about occupational exposure from co-workers' smoking. Your first search concept is the exposure. It can be represented by the MeSH headings OCCUPATIONAL EXPOSURE or ENVIRONMENTAL EXPOSURE. The second concept centers on co-workers' smoking. It can be represented by the phrase passive smoking. That concept maps to the MeSH heading TOBACCO SMOKE POLLUTION. You would then *AND* those concepts with the explosion of EPIDEMIOLOGIC STUDY CHARACTERISTICS. Table 4.7 shows the search strategy and a sample citation.

TABLE 4.7. Example of Search Strategy Formulation to Retrieve Citations on Etiology or Harm

Search question: What is the harm to you from a co-worker smoking?

1.   OCCUPATIONAL EXPOSURE
2.   ENVIRONMENTAL EXPOSURE
3.   1 *OR* 2
4.   3 *AND* EXPLODE EPIDEMIOLOGIC STUDY CHARACTERISTICS
6.   Limit to English

Authors	Coggins CR.
Title	A prospective study of passive smoking and coronary heart disease [letter; comment].
Comments	Comment on: Circulation 1997 May 20;95(10):2374-9
Source	Circulation. 97(18);1870-1; discussion 1872-3, 1998 May 12.
Major MeSH Headings	*Coronary Disease / et [Etiology] *Tobacco Smoke
MeSH headings	Cohort Studies Coronary Disease / ep [Epidemiology] Environmental Exposure Occupational Exposure/ Pollution / ae [Adverse Effects] Prospective Studies Questionnaires Risk Risk Factors United States / ep [Epidemiology]
MeSH Checktags	Female, Human, Male

Prognosis

The Evidence-Based Medicine searching techniques to retrieve quality citations on prognosis include using the subheadings MORTALITY and EPIDEMIOLOGY and the MeSH headings MORTALITY, MORBIDITY, and PROGNOSIS.

As an example, you have a search request to find out if the prognosis of someone with Lou Gehrig's Disease is improving. Your first search statement can include the phrase "Lou Gehrig," the word "ALS," and the MeSH heading AMYTROPHIC LATERAL SCLEROSIS, with the subheadings MORTALITY and EPIDEMIOLOGY: AMYTROPHIC LATERAL SCLEROSIS/EP, MO.

The second search statement would include the MeSH headings PROGNOSIS, MORTALITY, MORBIDITY, LIFE EXPECTANCY, and SURVIVAL. The third search statement would join the two search statements. The final search statement would limit to English language and HUMAN. Table 4.8 shows the sample search strategy, along with a sample citation.

When to Use Best-Evidence Techniques

Using the Evidence-Based Medicine searching techniques of attaching certain subheadings, including selected MeSH headings, and limiting to particular publication types will retrieve fewer, better-quality citations. The ultimate judge of which citations to print out is you. It is your search request based on your clinical question.

SUMMARY

This chapter has highlighted the popular free and fee-based MEDLINE searching systems available on the Internet at this moment, but the Internet changes every second. Searching systems can appear and disappear in a heartbeat. A recommendation is that you try several, then try to master a few different MEDLINE searching systems. Keep up with their enhancements. The MEDLINE searching systems you decide to use will be your personal decision, like picking ice cream flavors. Base your decision on your ease of

TABLE 4.8. Example of Search Strategy Formulation to Retrieve Quality Citations on Prognosis

Search question: Has the prognosis for Lou Gehrig's Disease improved?

1.   Lou Gehrig OR ALS OR AMYTROPHIC LATERAL SCLEROSIS/MO,EP
2.   PROGNOSIS OR MORBIDITY OR MORTALITY
3.   1 AND 2
4.   Limit to English, Human

Authors	Louwerse ES. Visser CE. Bossuyt PM. Weverling GJ.
Institution	Department of Neurology, Academic Medical Center, University of Amsterdam, The Netherlands.
Title	Amyotrophic lateral sclerosis: mortality risk during the course of the disease and prognostic factors. The Netherlands ALS Consortium.
Source	Journal of the Neurological Sciences. 152 Suppl 1:S10-7, 1997 Oct.
Major MeSH Headings	*Amyotrophic Lateral Sclerosis / mo [Mortality]
MeSH Headings	Age of Onset
	Age Factors
	Amyotrophic Lateral Sclerosis/ ge [Genetics]
	Amyotrophic Lateral Sclerosis / pp [Physiopathology]
	Disease Progression
	Follow-Up Studies
	Multivariate Analysis
	Netherlands / ep [Epidemiology]
	Prognosis
	Risk Factors
	Survival Analysis
MeSH Checktags	Aged, Female, Human, Male, Middle Age

Abstract

    We performed a historical cohort study of 307 untreated patients with probable or definite amyotrophic lateral sclerosis in order to investigate whether the mortality risk changed during the disease course and to identify prognostic factors at diagnosis. Patients were diagnosed in one of the academic hospitals in The Netherlands and followed up for at least 6 years after diagnosis. The median survival from diagnosis was 1.4 years (95% confidence interval, 1.3-1.6 years) with an estimated 5- and 10-year survival of 20 and 8%, respectively. Mortality was at its maximum in the second year after diagnosis and declined considerably thereafter. Observed mortality approached the expected mortality in patients who survived diagnosis 6 or more years. In univariate and multivariate analyses, young age, limb onset, and a long delay between initial weakness and diagnosis were associated with lower mortality. The better prognosis of limb onset patients was not observed in females. Patients with initial respiratory muscle weakness had the worst prognosis, with a median survival of only 2 months. The significantly greater mortality of older patients proved not to result from a rise in expected mortality only. In conclusion, the annual mortality risk in ALS does not remain constant throughout the disease and depends on age at diagnosis, site of onset, diagnostic delay, but also on the time since diagnosis. These findings may have consequences for the planning of symptomatic care and the design and analysis of therapeutic trials.

searching and your need for certain features. You can use any of the MEDLINE systems discussed here to perform a successful search, if you learn the nuances and features and master good searching techniques.

Be inquisitive. What MeSH headings, significant phrases, and words are included in your most relevant citations? Use those same MeSH headings, phrases, or words in additional search strategies and you may get more relevant results, again. If you have expertise in a subject area, trust your knowledge if you think the amount of citations you found is incorrect. Try to revise your search strategy. Notice if you get fewer or more citations than you expected.

If you retrieved more citations than you expected, here are some options to tighten your results. Choose a more exact MeSH heading or attach a subheading to a MeSH heading. Make your MeSH headings the central focus of the article. Filter for better-quality results. Limit to review articles, search for words or phrases in titles, or just narrow the number of years searched. If you retrieved fewer citations than you expected, consider exploding MeSH terms or removing a subheading. Try searching with other words or phrases or include more years in the number of years searched.

If you are still not satisfied with your search results, don't settle. Consult the MEDLINE searching system's cyber-help desk, a medical librarian, or your local librarian and use their expert searching suggestions. After all, the more you practice the searching techniques of the expert MEDLINE searchers, the closer you are to becoming an expert.

SELECTED BIBLIOGRAPHY

Anagnostelis, B. "Evaluation Criteria for Different Versions Of The Same Database—A Comparison of MEDLINE Services Available via the World Wide Web." Available: <http://omni.ac.uk/agec/iolim97/>. Accessed: 11 January 1999. Originally presented at Online Information 97: the 21st International Online Information Meeting, London, 9-11 December 1997.

"Criteria for Assessing the Quality of Health Information on the Internet." Available: <http://hitiweb.mitretek.org/docs/criteria.html>. Accessed: 11 January 1999.

Detmer, W.M. "MEDLINE on the Web: Ten Questions to Ask When Evaluating a Web Based Service." Available: <http://www.med.virginia. edu/~wmd4n/medline. html>. Accessed: 11 January 1999.

Engstrom, P. "MEDLINE Free-For-All Spurs Questions About Search Value, Who Pays." *Medicine on the Net* 2(Aug. 1996).

Eysenbach, G., and Diepgen, T.L. "Towards Quality Management of Medical Information on the Internet: Evaluation, Labelling, and Filtering of Information." *BMJ* 317(28 November 1998):1496-1502. Available: <http://www.bmj.com/cgi/content/full/317/7171/1496#art>. Accessed: 11 January 1999.

"Free MEDLINE on the Web: A Practical View." *Cyberpulse: Internet Tips for Health Science Research* 2 (Spring 1997). Available: <http://www.imr.on.ca/cyberpulse/no 2.htm>. Accessed: 11 January 1999.

Greenhalgh, T. "How to Read a Paper: The MEDLINE Database." BMJ 315(July 19, 1997). Available: <http://www.bmj.com/archive/7101/7101ed. htm#1-ref1>. Accessed: 11 January 1999.

Jacobs, M,; Edwards, A,; Graves, R,S.; and Johnson, E.D. "Criteria for Evaluating Alternative MEDLINE Search Engines." *Medical Reference Services Quarterly* 17(Fall 1998):1-12.

Malet, G. "MEDLINE." Available: <http://www._medmatrix.org/SPages/Medline. asp>. Accessed: 11 January 1999.

Mallen M. "Evaluating Search Engines: Task Force Progress Report. " *NAHRS (Nursing and Allied Health Resources Section) Newsletter* 18(March 1998):4,6-8.

Murphy, B. "Free MEDLINE Access: Why Pay?" (Position Paper). Available: <http://www.mc.duke.edu/mclibrary/limited/free_med.html>. Accessed: 11 January 1999.

Perry, H. "Dr. Felix's Free MEDLINE Page." Available: <http://www.docnet. org.uk/drfelix>. Accessed: 11 January 1999.

Sandlin, N. "What's the Deal with All This FREE MEDLINE?" *NETworking* (March 17, 1997). Available: <http://www.ama-assn.org/sci-pubs/amnews/net_97/nwkg0317.htm>. Accessed: 11 January 1999.

Chapter 5

Searching the Internet for Diseases

Alexa Mayo
Cynthia R. Phyillaier

INTRODUCTION

Searching for information on diseases is often serious business. Unlike searching for movie reviews or a recipe, searching for information about diseases carries a greater sense of urgency. For the consumer of health care, it can be intimidating, overwhelming, and frightening, especially if one is newly diagnosed. For the physician, even one experienced in computer searching, the maze of information on the Web can be equally overwhelming.

One of the core challenges of searching for information on disease is sorting through the many different types of information one can find. Information found on the Web relating to disease is a mix of the anecdotal, commercial, educational, and clinical. Searching for information about a disease on the Web often requires that one become familiar with body systems and with clinical language, concepts that consumers may never have had to explore. A second challenge of the Web is recognizing quality information.

Web searchers have a range of information needs. Some searchers are health practitioners with an interest in finding the answer to a specific, clinical question on which to base a patient care decision. They may be searching for a research article from a peer-reviewed publication or for a clinical practice guideline. Consumers may be interested in general information about a disease or in a health term. They may also be searching for clinical information with which to make informed decisions about their own care. Librarians must

77

know how to locate the full range of information about disease on the Web.

The enormous range of Internet resources relating to diseases includes practitioner-oriented clinical materials to patient/consumer information. Some sites are designed primarily for consumers, such as NOAH (http://www.noah.cuny.edu/); some specifically for physicians, such as CliniWeb (http://www.ohsu.edu/cliniweb/). Sites may include a range of information, with links on the page that separate (somewhat arbitrarily) the practitioner-oriented resources from the consumers', such as CancerNet (http://cancernet.nci.nih.gov/).

Much of the information on the Web is free and available to everyone. However, commercial vendors often do not provide free information to the public or to libraries. These commercial resources may be purchased by libraries and are made available only to their user community either via a password or through IP (Internet Protocol) verification. A link on the Web to a site does not guarantee its availability. Some sites require that one register as a user, but do not charge a fee to access the resource.

STARTING POINTS

Organizations, associations, foundations, institutions, societies, agencies, and clearinghouses often contain diverse resources under one roof. The missions of these groups are varied. Quality sites state their mission on the Web page, which would include the audience, either consumer or clinician, that they support. Some organizations serve both and may divide their resources with separate links to resources for the consumer or clinician.

Professional organizations may offer continuing medical education materials, notices about conferences and meetings, or meeting abstracts. Some publish books and offer a list of titles that can be ordered online; online journals published by the organization or association may also be available from the home page. Some professional organizations publish statements of care or clinical practice guidelines. The American Medical Association (http://www.ama-assn. org), the professional organization that is dedicated to the broad mission of promoting the "art and science of medicine and the betterment of public health,"[1] offers links to *JAMA* online, a list of publications for purchase, and other information.

Consumer-oriented organizations are aimed at providing patient support resources. They often provide educational materials, mailing lists, toll-free numbers, newsletters, support groups, and may include notification of national meetings related to specific diseases or conditions. Consumer sites usually provide information in nonclinical language. The American Cancer Society (http://www.cancer.org) offers information on cancer prevention, treatment, and survivorship. The Allergy and Asthma Network-Mothers of Asthmatics (AAN-MA) (http://www.aanma.org) offers a search feature with which to look up physicians affiliated with the AAN-MA. Also, many have brochures and fact sheets with the imprimatur of the organization, which helps to guarantee quality.

The National Institutes of Health (NIH) (http://www.nih.gov) and the National Health Council (http://www.spry.org/NHC.htm) both provide links to quality information. The NIH, one of the world's foremost biomedical research centers, is composed of a group of twenty-four smaller institutes, including the National Cancer Institute (http://www.nci.nih.gov) and the National Institute of Allergy and Infectious Diseases (NIAID) (http://www.niaid.nih.gov). The National Health Council is a nonprofit organization with links to nearly 100 health foundations and agencies, including the American Lung Foundation (http://www.lungusa.org), Arthritis Foundation (http://www.arthritis.org), and Lupus Foundation of America (http://www.lupus.org/lupus).

The Centers for Disease Control and Prevention (CDC) (http://www.cdc.gov), an agency of the Department of Health and Human Services, is dedicated to promoting "health and quality of life by preventing and controlling disease, injury, and disability."[2] The CDC includes eleven centers, institutes, and offices, including the National Center for Chronic Disease Prevention and Health Promotion, National Center for Environmental Health, Office of Genetics and Disease Prevention, National Center for HIV, STD, and TB Prevention, National Center for Infectious Diseases, and the Office of Global Health. From the CDC's home page, disease information is arranged alphabetically under the "Health Information" link. Resources obtained from the CDC are of excellent quality.

Medical gateway sites are excellent places to start to search for diverse disease information. They are committed to providing a range of resources—database searching, general information for the consumer, and research—all from within one site. NLM's consumer-oriented MEDLINEplus (http://medlineplus.nlm.nih.gov/medlineplus) contains a selected list of resources on disease arranged under "Health Topics." Preformulated MEDLINE searches that are narrowed to a particular aspect of the disease, such as diagnosis or treatment, link directly to the PubMed database. The Karolinska Institute (http://info.ki.se/ki) combines an alphabetic list of diseases and disorders, with an option to search for a disease that is not on the list, and also provides a link to search MEDLINE. Other sites that provide a gateway to disease information are HealthGate (http://www.healthgate.com), Medical Matrix (http://www.medmatrix.org), Healthfinder (http://www.healthfinder.org/default.htm), HealthWeb (http://healthweb.org/), CliniWeb (http://www.ohsu.edu/cliniweb/), Medsite Navigator (http://www.medsitenavigator.com/index.html), NOAH (http://www.noah.cuny.edu/), MedWeb (http://www.cc.emory.edu/WHSCL/medweb.html), Mayo Clinic Health Oasis, (http://www.mayohealth.org/), Hardin Meta Directory (http://www.lib.uiowa.edu/hardin/md/index.html), Medical World Search (http://www.mwsearch.com), and HealthAtoZ (http://www.HealthAtoZ.com).

WEB RESOURCES

Resources on disease are varied. The following are some of the types of information one can find on the Web.

Medical dictionaries or glossaries provide brief information about a disease, condition, or term. Definitions may include the body system of which the disease is a part, which would assist consumers in searching the more clinically oriented sources that organize resources by general type (autoimmune disease, kidney disease, infectious disease). "AMA's Medical Glossary" (http://www.ama-assn.org/ insight/ gen_glossary /glos_hm.htm) is aimed at the consumer. The "Michigan Electronic Library (MEL)" (http://mel.lib.mi.us/health/health-dictionaries.html) offers a list of health-related dictionaries and glossaries, some of which are devoted to specific diseases or conditions.

Directories provide brief information on a person, place, or thing. Medical-Net's "Hospital Select" (http://www.hospitalselect.com) is a reference source of information on individual hospitals in the United States; the "AMA Physician Select, On-Line Doctor Finder" (http://www.ama-assn.org/aps/amahg.htm) provides information about the specialists who would treat a specific disease.

Fact sheets/brochures/miscellaneous pamphlets, booklets, handouts, textbooks, monographs, news, research in progress, and assorted publications are authored by individuals, institutions, and companies. This group also includes personal testimonials, pitches for products by companies—such as pharmaceutical companies—and advertisements. "Diet and Arthritis Fact Sheet" is an informational sheet produced by the Arthritis Foundation (http://www.arthritis.org).

Database search systems are collections of data records that are organized by searchable fields such as author, title, and subject. Databases are often created and maintained by authoritative organizations, such as the National Library of Medicine (NLM) (http://www.nlm.nih.gov) or the National Cancer Institute (http://www.nci.nih.gov). Searching a database on diseases would almost always include a search of NLM's MEDLINE, the premier database in the field of medicine. MEDLINE uses a rich vocabulary to support searching for specific aspects of disease, such as etiology, diagnosis, and therapies. Searching MEDLINE is the best method of locating quality, peer-reviewed articles on a disease or condition. NLM's PubMed (http://www.ncbi.nlm.nih.gov/PubMed) and Internet Grateful Med (http://igm.nlm.nih.gov) both search the MEDLINE database (see Chapter 4 for more information about MEDLINE). Library collections are also databases.

Online journals/newsletters are of two general types: an online version of a print journal (*JAMA*, *Annals of Internal Medicine*, *BMJ*) and a journal that is only available on the Web, with no corresponding print version. Online journals are reliably obtained from the publisher's home page. However, online journals are also available from links within a database such as PubMed, from organized lists of online journals, and from diverse links throughout the Web. Current issues of online journals are more readily available than earlier years. Publishers such as the American Medical Association (http://www.ama-assn.org), for example, provide the full text of *JAMA* from 1996 to the present. Though somewhat dated, a collection of medical online journals and newsletters is available from Emory University's MedWeb (http://www.cc.emory/edu); a continually updated list of online journals and newsletters is available at New Jour (http://gort.ucsd.edu.newjour/). University of Texas M. D. Anderson Cancer Center: Medical Journals Online (http://www.mdacc.tmc.edu/~library/Mejoonln/MJOlinks.htm) and MedSite Navigator (http://www.medsitenavigator.com/med/A.html) maintain lists of online journals. Online journals are sometimes available only with a subscription.

Clinical practice guidelines provide a pathway to treating a particular disease or condition. They are "user-friendly statements that bring together the best external evidence and other knowledge necessary for decision making about a specific health problem."[3] These are authored by professional organizations such as the American College of Physicians (ACP) (http://www.acponline.org) or the Association of Health Care Policy and Research (AHCPR) (http://www.ahcpr.gov). Clinical practice guidelines primarily serve practitioners, and they may be collected from a variety of places. Guidelines without a date should not be considered useful. An example of a clinical guideline is "Guidelines for Laboratory Evaluation in the Diagnosis of Lyme Disease," published in ACP's Annals of Internal Medicine (http://www.acponline.org/journals/annals).

Clinical trials are experimental studies that investigate new drugs or treatments. Patients can, if they qualify, enroll in these experimental studies. A separate section within this chapter discusses clinical trials. CenterWatch Clinical Trials Listing Service (http://www.centerwatch.com) is a general listing of trials.

Online discussion lists and usenet newsgroups allow one to engage in online discussions about disease—either as someone living with a disease or as a caregiver. The interactivity of online discussion creates a forum for sharing information about disease, which includes emotional support. Online discussion lists and usenet newsgroups may be located in several ways. Liszt, The Mailing List Directory (http://www.Liszt.com), is a search tool that specializes in locating listservs—over 90,000 of them—and also provides search links to usenet newsgroups. Tile.Net (http://www.tile.net/lists/medicine.html) is a directory of listservs and usenet newsgroups. DejaNews (http://www.dejanews. com) provides access to usenet newsgroups. Web sites that are committed to providing all types of information—especially for the consumer—often contain an interactive link directly from the home page.

EVALUATING WEB RESOURCES

Materials obtained from the Web must be filtered or evaluated for quality and appropriateness. The labor involved in this process depends on how the information was retrieved. If a searcher knows of a reliable site, such as the CDC (http://www.cdc.gov), one can simply type in the Web address or uniform resource locator (URL), search the site, and obtain quality information. However, if one does not know of a specific, quality disease site, one must use a search tool, such as AltaVista (http://www.digital.altavista.com). Some search tools offer health information selectively, such as Medical Matrix (http://www.medmatrix.org/index.asp?) or HealthWeb (http://www.healthweb.org). In sites that gather information selectively, a higher quality of results can be expected, although not guaranteed.[4] Web pages or search tools that purport to provide high quality information may be rated or peer reviewed.

Although debate continues, sites may be considered of higher quality if they have been rated by an organization, such as Physician's Choice (http://www.mdchoice.com/instr.htm). Instruments and criteria used to rate health information have recently been shown to be inconsistent and uneven, which calls into question whether rating is useful or possible after all.[5] While the discussion concerning the rating of health information continues, it is best to use rated sites, with the caveat that the rating system may be questionable. Rated sites can generally be trusted, however, to separate anecdotal junk from potentially useful health information.

A resource on the Web that is peer reviewed indicates that the information has been scrutinized. Peer review in the traditional sense denotes that peers (experts) in the field have verified the information for completeness and accuracy. Peer review on the Web, however, may mean only that another person has evaluated the material. Although being peer reviewed does not guarantee quality, it is another imperfect method of separating the anecdotal from the potentially useful.

Searchers for information on disease must assess the information themselves, as resources on the Web can be dangerously unreliable. A recent study of the quality of information relating to the study of childhood diarrhea illustrated that only 20 percent of articles published by traditional medical sources on the Web contained information that conformed to current American Academy of Pediatrics (AAP) guidelines for management of acute diarrhea.[6] Information from major academic institutions did not improve the likelihood of compliance. Medical information, even from peer-reviewed, rated, or academic sites, should be critically evaluated to judge its credibility. Criteria or quality standards can be applied to Web resources to help establish reliability.[7] These criteria are content, authority/authorship, currency, and design/ease-of-use.

Content

References for all sources of content should be listed. If primary sources are used, the data source or method of collecting data should be revealed. The linked sites should be stable and of quality.

Authority/Authorship

The authoring body should be clearly stated, with an address and a method of contact. Online journals should list the editorial board; the mission of the page should be clearly stated. Financial relationships, including underwriting, advertising, and relationship to sponsors, should be disclosed. The authoring body should be dependable, as in a government or academic site.

Currency

Production date and revision date should be listed. Linked sites should also be current.

Design/Ease of Use

The information should be presented in an easy-to-follow manner, without unnecessary clutter. Graphics should be relevant to the content of the page; any special features should enhance the mission of the page.

SEARCHING FOR COMMON DISEASES

There is no single best way to search for disease information on the Web. Some diseases are high profile and prevalent, generate public interest, and may have considerable research funding. These types of diseases (AIDS, asthma, cancer, diabetes, etc.) may have their own associations, foundations, or even institute. Medical search tools' indexes and menus contain links to common diseases. Other disease types may be more difficult to locate on the Web. These would include rare diseases, those which may be perceived as not affecting the general population, and those which do not generate serious research dollars. Diseases that are difficult to fit into one disease category and emerging diseases and therapies may also be difficult to locate. One must alter search techniques depending on the disease.

A search for information about a disease begins by looking at any known sites of quality on the subject. For more information, consult general medical sites that specialize in organizing and providing information. A disease such as cancer is well represented on the Web. Illustrating how one might search for cancer information using selected medical sites demonstrates universal concepts and methods for searching the Web.

As a common disease, it is not surprising that there are quality sites on the Web devoted entirely to cancer: Oncolink (http://www.oncolink.upenn.edu/) and CancerNet (http://cancernet.nci.nih.gov/) are two of these sites. Oncolink allows one to find information from several perspectives. Its home page provides a variety of selections, ranging from "Disease Oriented Menus," "Medical Specialty Oriented Menus," and "Clinical Trials," to "Psychosocial Support and Personal Experiences." The home page also contains a link to "Search Oncolink" for those who would rather not wade through a variety of menus. The site is maintained by the University of Pennsylvania Cancer Center and there are links from the home page ("About OncoLink," "Editorial Board") that clearly state where the posted information originates.

The National Cancer Institute's (NCI's) CancerNet defines its audience as falling into one of three groups: "Patients and the Public," "Health Professionals," and "Basic Researchers." Although anyone can search all of the information, this division shows the depth and variety of resources that are available. There are useful sheets that describe the site ("About CancerNet") and CANCER-LITR, NCI's bibliographic database. CANCERLITR is relatively easy to search: entered terms map to articles with correct Medical Subject Headings (MeSH) terminology, so that if "lung cancer" is entered, articles on "lung neoplasms" are retrieved. Although one may not need to know the medical terminology to access information, this site does require a substantial amount of medical sophistication to comprehend the areas other than those found in the "Patients and the Public" section.

Sites other than those devoted solely to cancer may also contain valuable and authoritative information on the disease. Medical Matrix (http://www.medmatrix.org/index.asp?), for instance, states that its "target audience is primarily United States physicians and health care workers who are on the front line in prescribing treatment for disease conditions."[8] It uses a menu format of disease categories and has several major strengths: it ranks sites (criteria are posted), it is peer reviewed (by the professional editorial board), and listed entries are annotated. Cancer can be searched by selecting the menu choice "Oncology" or by entering search terms for the type of cancer information needed. Entering the term "lung cancer" retrieves items organized under the "Oncology" and "Pulmonology" sections. Particularly useful are links to "Lung Tumors Multidisciplinary Database," located at University of Iowa College of Medicine's Virtual Hospital (http://www.vh.org/) and the "NCI CancerLit Database on Lung Cancer"(http://www.gretmar.com/webdoctor/OncologyCCLung.html). As might be expected in a site designed for health professionals, it will probably yield the most meaningful results for members of this group. It can be useful, however, for motivated consumers who take the time to familiarize themselves with medical terminology in order to obtain in-depth information on a subject.

Quality information also can be found at healthfinder (http://www.healthfinder.org/default.htm). Healthfinder has a variety of menu lists on its home page, in addition to a search box for entering a search term or disease. The site's selection policy, which is fully set forth, clearly indicates that the searcher should expect primarily information from U.S. government agencies; national voluntary, nonprofit, and professional organizations; and academic institutions and libraries. Since cancer is one of the "hot topics" choices on the home page, one can locate cancer information directly from this link. Another alternative is to use the search box to enter a term such as "lung cancer." This query retrieved twenty-three items that were broken down into the categories "Web resources" and "organizations." The majority of the resources were U.S. government (e.g., "CDC Prevention Guidelines for Cigarette Smoking and Lung Cancer"), but there was also a link to Oncolink. Since this site is primarily aimed at consumers, medical terminology is not the barrier it can be at sites established for medical professionals.

HealthWeb (http://healthweb.org/) covers information on the spectrum of diseases, including cancer. It was designed and is maintained by a cooperative of major academic institutions in the Midwest. All resources and links are evaluated and selected by librarians, and choices are made with both health professionals and consumers in mind. Search results are displayed with the best sites listed first; these are indicated by a number of stars. A search of the term "lung cancer" retrieved ninety-one matches; the first linked to Oncolink. Other links in the first ten items retrieved were "MedWeb: Oncology," "Ask NOAH About: Cancer," and "NCI/PDQ Cancer News," all excellent sites.

NLM's MEDLINEplus (http://medlineplus.nlm.nih.gov/medlineplus/) presents information in a different manner. Although it contains a search screen that permits typing in a search term, it also has a small (but growing) list of "Health Topics." There are three topics related to cancer on the current list: "Breast Cancer," "Cancer (General)," and "Prostate Cancer." To locate information on lung cancer, either type the term into the search entry form or view the "Cancer (General)" choices. The first option (using the search form), for this topic, is less than satisfactory, since it only retrieves two items— one a clearinghouse and the other an organization. The second option provides excellent information, even though there are no direct links to the term "lung cancer." It provides links to PubMed for searching the MEDLINE database and a link to appropriate cancer definitions (e.g., lung neoplasms). Sites with links are arranged by categories so it is clear which information is coming from the NLM and the NIH and which information is coming from other governmental and organizational sources.

Cliniweb (http://www.ohsu.edu/cliniweb/), a site established by medical and information specialists at Oregon Health Sciences University, is designed for health practitioners and students. It is organized according to the MeSH disease and anatomy classifications and links to the PubMed database. In addition, there are links to numerous academic and governmental sites. It provides useful information, as long as one knows to look for "neoplasms" or "carcinoma" when searching for information on cancer. Consumers would probably find MEDLINEplus more user friendly. For the intended audience, health practitioners, this site can provide a number of pathways for retrieving information on medical subjects.

Two sites specifically oriented toward consumers that provide excellent coverage of information are "NOAH: New York Online Access to Health" (http://www.noah.cuny.edu/) and "Mayo Clinic Health Oasis" (http://www.mayohealth.org/). NOAH is a unique collaboration of state, local, and federal resources; the content is selected by contributing editors, all of whom are library science professionals. NOAH's list of "Health Topics" includes broad subjects that are then narrowed in scope once they are selected. Cancer is covered in several broad categories, including definitions, care and treatment, and lists of information resources. Cancer types can be accessed by selecting the letter of an alphabetical list, or they can be searched by keyword or concept using the site's search engine. Although only two listings are under the term "lung cancer," both link to the PDQ database at the National Cancer Institute's Cancer-Net site. These particular PDQ resources may be problematic for consumers, NOAH's intended audience, as they are identified as coming from the part of PDQ "for physicians."

The "Mayo Clinic Health Oasis" is another excellent source of information for consumers. Editors of the site consist of physicians at the Mayo Clinic, and special emphasis is placed on providing timely information, with revision dates noted. Nine major centers are listed on the home page; "Cancer" is one of them. Secondary choices include an extensive list of reference articles, a cancer glossary, and a section titled "Ask the Mayo Physician." Similar to NOAH, this site has entries for lung cancer on its list of reference articles. However, these are all articles written by Mayo Clinic staff (e.g., "You may have a role in your risk for this disease"). A notable distraction of the site, which is not present on the sites previously discussed, is commercial advertisements (primarily by pharmaceutical companies). Although they have been relegated to the top and right sides of the Web pages, they can be obtrusive.

The Hardin Meta Directory of Internet Health (http://www.lib.uiowa.edu/hardin/md/index.html) describes itself as a "list of lists" and is organized in a manner that is most useful for health professionals and information specialists. Its home page displays a number of large, medium, and small lists for each medical area. Connection rates of links included in the Hardin Meta Directory are checked and updated on a regular basis so the user can be assured that information is current. One must know that cancer will be found under the "Oncology" entry, since there is no search entry form; selecting this leads to sixteen large, three medium, and one small list on the subject.

SEARCHING FOR LESS COMMON DISEASES

Many diseases are not as common as cancer but are still relatively prevalent. These diseases are typically ones that are not listed as separate menu items on major medical Web sites. Diseases may be listed under broader or related topics; therefore, a knowledge of medical terminology is helpful when deciding which category to search. It may be necessary to search these sites by entering specific search terms. To supplement information using these methods, the next step would be to search for the disease using general search tools (search engines/directories). Search tools, however, when used to search for diseases, typically retrieve too much information, including much extraneous data. It is therefore important that the searcher be familiar with search techniques used (see Chapter 2) in order to narrow and focus the information retrieved.

Lyme disease is a good example of a disease that falls into this group and for this reason can be used to demonstrate methods needed for searching lesser-known disease entities. In searching for Lyme disease information at the selected Web sites previously searched for cancer information, it is interesting to note the similar and also different techniques needed to obtain useful information. Consumer-oriented sites tend to have more links to diseases with their everyday names (rather than scientific or medical) and are often the easiest for locating initial information. Frequently, these sites lead to the appropriate medical terminology, which assists the searcher in locating additional information. Sites will be addressed in order of the easiest to the most difficult for locating information on Lyme disease. Retrieval techniques in a few major search engines will then be examined.

Only one of the sites previously examined for cancer information (NOAH) contains a menu item for Lyme disease. A very lengthy section on Lyme disease displayed on the "Health Topics List" provides links to just about every site on the Web with credible information on the subject. Since it is consumer oriented, and provides information bilingually (English and Spanish), it is an excellent site for consumers to consult on the subject.

Healthfinder, since it is also a consumer-oriented site, provides quick and easy access to quality information for the nonprofessional. By entering the term "Lyme disease," four "organizations" and eleven "Web resources," including "Consumer Health Information, National Institutes of Health," are retrieved.

MEDLINEplus is useful for locating information on Lyme disease. Although Lyme disease is currently not one of the subjects listed on the "Health Topics" page, one can click on a link to the MEDLINE database and search for information in that database. Even if the searcher does not know the scientific term for Lyme disease (*Borrelia burgdorferi* infection), typing "Lyme disease" in the subject search area of the database retrieves over 4,000 articles on the subject, focused by subheading.

The Mayo Clinic Health Oasis does not have a separate center for Lyme disease at its site, as it did for cancer, so it is necessary to enter the term "Lyme disease" in the search entry form. This technique retrieves twenty-three items with links, all of them from the Mayo Organization, and they include information on a variety of subjects such as tick bites, vaccine studies, and a link to library references on infectious diseases.

Medical Matrix does not contain an obvious category in which Lyme disease would be found, but the search form allows one to enter the term, with a number of excellent results. Since the site is aimed at health professionals, they can locate particular aspects of diseases here and results fall within one of several categories: infectious diseases, pediatrics, or rheumatology. Links are to a dosing table from the American College of Physicians, Pediatric Clinical Practice Guidelines at the Canadian Medical Association, and several pamphlets on Lyme disease from the Centers for Disease Control and Prevention.

CliniWeb can be searched two ways for Lyme disease. One can "Browse" through the MeSH hierarchical listing of diseases, or one can select "Search" by entering "Lyme disease" in the search form. The second method is much easier for most consumers and it leads to an appropriate term for the disease (*Borrelia* Infections). Included here is a list of links to a number of quality sites with information on Lyme disease (CDC, Harvard University, American College of Physicians) and a link to the PubMed database for preconfigured searches on the subject. Health care professionals may prefer to search by medical subject headings to retrieve particular information about Lyme disease, and this site has that capability.

There are two methods for retrieving information on Lyme disease from HealthWeb. The alphabetical subject list does not have a broad category for "diseases" or a specific one for "Lyme disease." There are menu selections for "Infectious Diseases" and "Rheumatology"; in this instance, if one follows the rheumatology link, it leads to a list of rheumatic disease resources that includes the treatment guidelines of the American College of Rheumatology. This method would likely be used by health professionals who are familiar with the terminology and medical classifications. The second method for retrieving information is by typing the term "Lyme disease" in the search entry form; this yields thirty documents, including one titled "Managing Lyme Disease" and several from the MedWeb site at Emory University.

Since the Hardin Meta Directory is a "list of lists," all of them in medical terminology, it would be fairly tedious to search and successfully locate information on Lyme disease without a medical background. Those with the background can find information by selecting individual categories (e.g., Rheumatology, Microbiology and Infectious Diseases) that they feel will be relevant. They can then select and examine the individual Web sites that interest them. Individuals without the specialized knowledge required by this site would do better to either search one of the other sites mentioned in this section or to use a search engine.

Search tools (search engines or search directories) can be useful in supplementing information on diseases obtained from the medical sites previously mentioned. There are a couple of provisos: search engines should be selected with care, *at least* two different search engines/directories should be searched, and it is important to become familiar with the "rules" for searching them (see Chapter 2).

Yahoo! (http://www.yahoo.com) is an excellent place to begin. Unlike the majority of search tools, this directory site has been reviewed by people. For that reason, links from the menu option often lead to quality retrieval. To search Lyme disease using the menu, link to the broad category "Health" and the subcategory "Diseases and Conditions." "Lyme Disease" is a menu choice that links to a number of quality sites, including NOAH, the CDC site on Lyme disease, and the "Lyme Disease Information Resource," a clearinghouse for information that has many useful links. Yahoo also provides a search engine option for those who prefer to search this way. Typing "Lyme disease" retrieves the sites previously obtained from the menu search and a number of additional commercial sites that advertise products. To be effective in narrowing the search, reading the "Help" section assists in obtaining the best results. Use the "rules" of the search engine (+"lyme disease") to search and retrieve the category matches for Lyme disease and its related organizations as before.

Hotbot (http://www.hotbot.com) is a search tool without a menu. Instead, it offers a powerful search feature. Entering "Lyme disease" without any restrictions results in the computer "robot" of the search engine returning all sites where those two words appear together (15,240 Web matches). The strength of HotBot is in its capability of allowing the searcher to narrow a search by choosing restrictions. There are a number of ways to limit a search, for example, by language, domain, date, or Web page depth. By limiting the "Lyme disease" search to only English, sites from January 1,

1998 to the present, by the domains .edu, .gov, or .org, and to only the top or front page of Web sites, the search retrieves 1,228 Web matches. There are even more specific ways to limit the search, but this technique is indicative of what can be done with this search engine to locate quality Web sites. Although many of the less helpful sites are eliminated by limiting a search, it still remains essential to assess the retrieved sites. Search results in HotBot are ranked and displayed from the highest to lowest levels.

AltaVista (http://www.altavista.com) is another large search engine that performs computerized searching on entered search terms. Unlike Hotbot, it currently does not have as many ways to limit searches, but it does provide the capability to "Refine Your Search" using a list of related subjects/terms. AltaVista allows the searcher to require relevant topics and exclude ones not applicable. Entering +"Lyme disease" in the search entry form results in 16,243 retrieved Web pages. Refining the search by requiring that the words "lyme" and "infection" be present narrows the results to 5,004. Web sites located by this search engine are not ranked, so one must often browse and evaluate multiple sites before obtaining useful ones.

SEARCHING FOR RARE AND EMERGING DISEASES

The approach in searching for information about a rare or emerging disease is the same as with any disease: go directly to a quality site if one is known, for instance, the National Center for Infectious Diseases (NCID) (http://www.cdc.gov/ncidod/) or World Health Organization: Communicable Disease Surveillance and Response (http://www.who.int/emc). One may also browse using the menu option of one of the medical search sites. Rare and emerging diseases, however, will most likely not be listed on directory menus. The next option is to use any search feature that is available on the general medical sites page, which searches the contents of the page. If no resources are available, then the searcher must use general search engines to obtain resources (see Chapter 2). Searching for a rare disease in several search engines and in a metasearch engine will illustrate the techniques for searching.

Binswanger's disease is a rare disease that does not appear on the disease menus of any of the medical sites. Therefore, it is appropriate to search very broadly, using a large search engine. A search in AltaVista (http://www.altavista.com) for "Binswanger's Disease" (in quotes) yielded thirty-seven items. Many of the links were useless: dead links, listserv messages from 1995 and 1996, a textbook advertisement, a résumé for a physician, and a list of paper sessions for a 1995 international conference. Among the outdated and useless items, however, were links to the National Institute of Neurological Disorders and Stroke (NINDS) (http://www.ninds.nih.gov), part of NIH and the National Organization for Rare Disorders (NORD) (http://www.rarediseases.org). Both sites provide useful information on the disease, including a definition, synonyms, information about treatments, prognosis, and where to obtain more information.

A search in HotBot (http://www.hotbot.com) for the same disease yielded forty-seven items. The results were much the same as AltaVista's. Again, there were many useless items, including resources that only mentioned Binswanger's disease but did not provide any content. Both NINDS and NORD, quality resources, appeared on the list of resources found by HotBot. For specific information about a rare disease such as Binswanger's disease, it would also be beneficial to search PubMed for research articles.

In searching for rare diseases, the challenge is often in obtaining retrieval. This contrasts with the usual challenge of the Web—limiting retrieval, or how not to find too much information. One method of searching for an obscure disease is to use a metasearch engine, such as Dogpile (http://dogpile.com) or Profusion (http://www.profusion.com). These engines search multiple search tools simultaneously.

Dogpile is a metasearch engine that allows one to search up to twenty-four search tools at the same time. Dogpile lists the twenty-four tools on its "Custom Search" page and allows the searcher to pick the tools to search and the order in which they display. Entering the terms "binswanger's disease" in the search form on the main page results in a display of Web sites grouped by the search engine. Search tools return different results because they each search the Web differently: Yahoo! produced none, Lycos listed forty-one, and Excite Web Search produced 104. The total number of items that the search tool found is displayed, although only the first ten resources appear. There is a link to see all of the results located by that search tool. The Dogpile search located the NINDS and NORD resources, along with many more, requiring the searcher to evaluate the retrieval carefully.

Search engines and metasearch engines can also be of particular value in providing access to information on emerging diseases and therapies and alternative medicine (see Chapter 6, on consumer health, and Chapter 7, on alternative medicine). The Web provides an international forum for discussion and collaboration. One can read about non-FDA-approved drugs that are being used outside of the United States, drug trials in other countries, infectious diseases that are most prevalent overseas, studies that are in the preliminary stages (prepublication), or material from newsletters and nonrefereed journals. The Web also provides access to naturopaths, whose expertise would not be generally available in the mainstream medical literature. Selected sites are devoted to emerging diseases and alternative medicine (see Chapter 7); use search engines or metasearch engines to search most comprehensively.

SEARCHING FOR OPEN CLINICAL TRIALS

A logical extension of seeking information on a chronic or potentially terminal disease often includes a search for current clinical trials. This is primarily done by health professionals and information specialists, although some databases, such as those aimed at patients with AIDS or rare diseases, recruit directly. Since most clinical trials have specific inclusion criteria, a physician referral is almost always required.

Initially, the majority of clinical trials on the Web were for cancer patients (NCI's CancerTrials, http://cancertrials.nci.nih.gov/) or AIDS patients (Clinical Trials Information Service, http://www.actis.org/actihome.html). A number of specialized sites and databases (CANCERLIT, AIDSLINE) deal only with a particular disease entity. However, within the past several years, general sites on the Web have been developed that include open clinical trials on a variety of diseases. In addition, many more general medical sites offer links to clinical trials.

Consumers may not know what defines a clinical trial. Quality consumer-oriented sites, such as NOAH, provide information about clinical trials in terms that are understandable. Clinical trials attempt to answer specific questions about treating diseases—either with new drugs or agents or by using established treatments in a new manner. Open clinical trials are those recruiting new patients to study, whereas closed trials no longer accept new patients. Clinical trials generally fall into one of four major categories: Phase I, Phase II, Phase III, or Adjuvant studies. Each clinical trial has a protocol, or a "set of rules" by which the study is conducted.

Phase I studies are used to determine if a new treatment can be given safely. If a drug is involved, the trial participants may be divided into groups and different doses of the drug given to each group. Phase I trials determine if a drug has efficacy in the disease being treated and whether it causes harmful side effects. For this reason, Phase I trials generally are only offered to patients for whom all conventional therapy has failed, since there is no guarantee of efficacy and there can be considerable risk.

Phase II trials build on the results of Phase I trials; slightly larger groups are enrolled in the protocol, and the primary goal is to determine efficacy. Phase III studies are further extensions of Phase II trials; they are usually compared to the standard treatment for the disease. In this trial group, the people receiving the standard treatment are called the "control" group.

Adjuvant studies are used primarily with patients who have had cancer and had their disease surgically removed. These are treatments in addition to surgery that attempt to improve the patients' chances for a cure for their disease.

CenterWatch Clinical Trials Listing Service (http://www.centerwatch.com) is an excellent beginning point for locating clinical trials, as it contains trials for many diseases. It is searchable by disease categories, and all of the trials listed are open (enrolling new patients). After locating a disease entity, one may narrow the listings by geographic area. The site is sponsored by pharmaceutical companies.

It is important to search more than one clinical trial site to determine all options. There is no one resource, for instance, that lists every clinical trial, since many individual medical centers and companies offer trials. To locate clinical trials, consider using a search engine (such as HotBot) that allows for narrowing retrieved sites by domain name, so that the search can be limited to academic medical centers or governmental sites. Search for "clinical trials" and the specific disease. Using a broad search engine without limiting retrieval would result in a comprehensive search, but search results could require considerable time to assess. A comprehensive search would locate commercial sites, such as trials sponsored by pharmaceutical companies.

After locating sites with a specific disease entity, it is important to determine if the clinical trials listed are currently open. In addition, sites that allow limiting by geographic area are very useful. Some clinical trial sites list eligibility and exclusion criteria extensively, whereas others may only list a contact person and telephone number or address. Finally, it is important that patients discuss trials in which they are interested with their physicians to determine if the trials are appropriate for their particular condition. Even the best clinical trial sites can provide seemingly erroneous leads if the patient misinterprets them or does not meet the eligibility criteria.[9]

CONCLUSION

The immediate challenge of applying disease information obtained from the Web is to provide consistent, quality information, both to consumers and to physicians. Some excellent sites make searching for disease information, especially for common diseases, very straightforward. For rarer diseases, this becomes more difficult and requires that one use a search engine or metasearch engine. One must become aware of the search engine's capabilities and features to obtain the very best information. As the Web grows, debate will continue on how to deliver quality information without inhibiting the open and lively sharing of information that characterizes the Web.

REFERENCE NOTES

1. American Medical Association—Mission Statement. Available: <http://www.ama.org/about/mission.htm>. Accessed: 17 November 1998.

2. About CDC—CDC Mission. Available: <http://www.cdc.gov/aboutcdc.htm>. Accessed: 13 November 1998.

3. Clinical Practice Guideline—Introduction. Available: <http:itsa.ucsf.edu/~petsam/intor.html>. Updated: October 12,22,29. Accessed: 4 November 1998.

4. Lindberg, D.A.B. and Humphreys, B.L. "Medicine and Health on the Internet: The Good, the Bad, and the Ugly." *JAMA* 280(October 21, 1998):1303-4.

5. Jadad, A.R. and Gagliardi, A. "Rating Health Information on the Internet: Navigating to Knowledge or to Babel?" *JAMA* 279(February 25, 1998):611-4.

6. McClung, H.J.; Murray, R.D.; and Heitlinger, L.A. "The Internet As a Source for Current Patient Information [Electronic article]. *Pediatrics* 1998;101(6):e2. Accessed: 30 October 1998.

7. Silberg, W.M.; Lundberg, G.D.; and Musaccio, R.A. "Assessing, Controlling, and Assuring the Quality of Medical Information on the Internet: Caveant Lector et Viewor—Let the Reader and Viewer Beware." *JAMA* 277(April 16, 1997):1244-5.

8. Medical Matrix. Available: <http://www.medmatrix.org/info/about.html>. Accessed: 29 October 1998.

9. Jeffrey, N.A.. "A Little Knowledge." *The Wall Street Journal*, October 19, 1998, p. R8.

Chapter 6

Consumer Health Information on the Internet

Janet M. Coggan

INTRODUCTION

As consumers in the 1990s became more sensitized to health issues and health insurance companies imposed more constraints on the individual's access to health care providers, the availability of consumer health and patient education information exploded. The problem for consumers is *not* in finding information. There exists almost *too* much information. The problem lies in locating accurate, high-quality information that will be of use to the consumer. This has proven especially true with the rising popularity of the Internet and the World Wide Web. Many computer users have "surfed the Net" and gone on the "information superhighway." Vast amounts of medical and health information exist on the Internet. As Eysenbach and Diepgen recently observed:

> There has been explosive growth in recent years of the Internet and World Wide Web as tools for seeking and communicating health and medical information, with increasing numbers of physicians and health care institutions maintaining Web sites.[1]

Because any computer can retrieve at least *some* information from Internet sites on consumer health topics, it has become fashionable to believe that anyone can succeed in searching, despite having no search skills. However, it is not so simple, as many librarians will attest, to retrieve a few, highly relevant pieces of information on a specific topic. Becoming a skilled literature database searcher requires special training, certain intellectual processes, logical thinking, and specific strategies to initiate a thorough search on any database, much less on an unregulated entity such as the Internet. The problem-solving process of surveying the lay literature is far more complex than the average computer user imagines. This is compounded by the fact that anyone can retrieve instant hits from the Internet, using one of the many search engines currently available. Because unskilled searchers can come up with an answer to a question, although it may not be the *best* or even the *correct* answer, many individuals are satisfied. This lays the foundation for the spread of inaccurate health information from the Internet and the World Wide Web. Such inaccurate information can very rapidly become disseminated and may negatively affect a patient's health if taken as truthful data. The potential for harm is very real.

SEARCHING THE INTERNET

The issue thus becomes finding *good* information after formulating a strategy that takes into account all the factors in searching a particular topic. One of the first considerations should focus on the language used in the search request. Databases, by and large, take advantage of a controlled vocabulary, or thesaurus, to use in the search question. The Internet, however, offers no such availability. Computer users frequently use whatever words they can think of to search a topic. The keyword search, as opposed to the controlled vocabulary search, is far less efficient in terms of specific retrieval. Although the number of patients using the Internet to retrieve information on their condition is increasing, patients tend to use nonmedical terms to describe and search for information on their condition.[2] Rose and colleagues state that access to reliable and valid World Wide Web sites should be provided for patients who express an interest in searching the Internet for medical information. It helps for the searcher to consider very carefully the language used in an Internet search. It also helps to take advantage of the Boolean connectors "and," "or," and "not." These connectors, when used to link similar terms, such as cancer *or* neoplasm, can significantly affect the outcome of an Internet retrieval.

An additional consideration concerns the specific Internet site one chooses to search. Although using a search engine may yield fruitful information, a searcher may also go directly to any site and search. Many universities, associations, and professional journals have World Wide Web sites available for users to search. Professionally produced materials usually have undergone some measure and degree of peer review, have been assessed in terms of the quality of content and the impact on users, and have been subjected to comparison with evidence to determine accuracy. Using certain criteria, such as authorship, attribution of research data, disclosure of references, and currency of information, consumers can judge for themselves if the site provides credible and useful data. Timeliness must form a major criterion for evaluating information retrieved from the Internet. This becomes relatively simple to determine because most World Wide Web pages have dates on them reflecting the last time information was entered. Please refer to Chapter 3, "Megasites for Health Care Information," for more in-depth data on consumer-oriented Internet sites.

As for the issue of reliable sites, the phenomenon has not escaped the attention of those designing sites for the Internet. As Donald Lindberg and Betsy Humphreys remark:

> To highlight reliable content, health sciences libraries and other organizations are producing directories of Internet-accessible health information emanating from sources they consider to be dependable and useful for selected user groups.[3]

Lindberg and Humphreys suggest that individuals could utilize well-organized directory sites and achieve more complete results in a shorter period of time for their searches. They also recommend using sites that are regularly updated to avoid the problems of changes in content.[3]

An additional criterion must include how easily users can locate the relevant material within the site once they find it. If users must scroll through page after page to find appropriate information on their specific topic, they quickly become frustrated. This frequently occurs on consumer health and patient information sites, as so many topics may be available. The design of the World Wide Web site therefore becomes a key issue for evaluation. It is all too easy for users to become overwhelmed by a site with poor-quality information. Consumers need to judge if the data they retrieve contain useful information to assist them in making informed decisions about the specific health issue.

The volume of information on the Internet can be daunting to any consumer. Eng and colleagues note that "the volume of information on the World Wide Web is so vast that even the best search engines have cataloged only about 28 percent of it."[4] Much of that information is, as the authors point out, "health related and researching health information is one of the most popular reasons for using the Internet." Eng and colleagues note that health information is now more quickly accessible than ever before and answers to almost all questions are readily available. It may be that the growth of the Internet will lead to a transfer from the traditional health professional as the purveyor of knowledge to a more patient- and consumer-centered method of health decision making.[4] Eng and colleagues further suggest that many factors contribute to this evolution, including patients' higher level of interest in details of their personal health care, the explosion of health care information and concomitant inability of individual clinicians to stay current, the emphasis on health care promotion and disease prevention, the aging of the general population, and the interest in alternative health care treatments.[4]

INTERNET OPTIONS

Many options are available for searchers to use, including bulletin boards, electronic journals, mailing lists, professional association and organization sites, individual university sites, self-help or support groups, and newsgroups, to mention only a few. A basic consideration for many consumers is how to determine where to go first for information. This determination will rest on the topic the searcher wants to search. For example, if consumers want data on heart disease, it might prove beneficial to look at the American Heart Association World Wide Web site at <http://www.americanheart.org>; or they could go to a medical center such as the Mayo Clinic at <http://www.mayohealth.org>; or to a health sciences library at a university, such as the University of Florida Health Science Center

Library at <http://www.library.health.ufl.edu>; or to a site such as the Virtual Hospital, which includes the *Iowa Health Book* at <http://www. vh.org>; or to a site such as Ask Dr. Weil at <http://cqi. pathfinder. com/drweil>, where specific questions may be answered from the database, which pertains to home remedies and natural medicine and emphasizes self-care. Please refer to Chapter 7 on alternative medicine for discussion of nontraditional options for consumers. If a user finds it preferable to locate an online support or self-help group on a specific help topic, that option is available through a site such as healthfinder at <http://www.healthfinder. gov>, a gateway to a consumer health and human services information site from the U.S. government.

INTERNET SITES

Consumers searching for health information on the Internet generally look for topics among the leading causes of death for women and men. According to the World Health Organization, in 1966, the leading causes of death for women were heart disease, cancer, stroke, lower respiratory infections, mental disorders, diabetes, chronic pulmonary disease, nephritis, and chronic liver disease. For men, the leading causes of death were cancer, heart disease, stroke, accidents, chronic pulmonary disease, lower respiratory infections, mental disorders, suicide, chronic liver disease, and diabetes.[5]

Although consumers will seek information on disease, the highly technical terminology may present comprehension barriers. Of course, many strategies will accomplish information retrieval, but as a medical librarian, this author favors first going to a site such as the American Medical Association Health Insight at <http://www. ama-assn.org/consumer.htm>. Scanning the health information containing articles on specific medical conditions will yield data on the topics previously listed as the leading causes of death. In addition, this site has an atlas of the human body and a medical glossary to consult when the vocabulary needs explanation. After viewing the AMA site, moving to a more specific collection of information, such as the full text of *The Columbia University College of Physicians and Surgeons Complete Home Medical Guide*, located at <http:// cpmcnet.columbia.edu/tests/guide/>, might prove of use. Visiting a medical library, such as the one of selected Internet resources at Yale University at <http://www.med.yale.edu/library/sir/>, may offer valuable data under the consumer health portion of the site. If a consumer wanted to review support group options, he or she could go to <http://www.dejanews.com/> and consult the *alt.support* newsgroup hierarchy for an extensive list. Should the consumer want to determine a potential physician experienced in treating the specific health condition, he or she could go to the Best Doctors site at <http://www.bestdoctors.com/> and find information about specialists in the preferred geographic area. If the condition is rare or in an advanced stage of development, the consumer may want to review the clinical trials by disease categories available at CenterWatch, <http://www.centerwatch.com/studies/>, for possible participation. If the consumer wants to retrieve information from a biomedical database such as MEDLINE, the HealthGate site at <http://www.healthgate.com/>, among others, provides free access to many of the National Library of Medicine databases and also contains a non-NLM database with information on diagnostic procedures. Should information on pharmaceutical products be desired, the HealthSquare site at <http://www.healthsquare.com> offers the full text of the *Physicians Desk Reference (PDR) Family Guide to Prescription Drugs*, the *PDR Family Guide to Women's Health*, and the *PDR Family Guide Encyclopedia of Medical Care*. If a consumer has specific questions not answered by any of these sites, Net Wellness at <http://www.netwellness.org> features a section called "Ask an Expert," which has a question and answer option. This strategy is but one alternative for a consumer wanting to retrieve health information from the Internet.

EVALUATING INTERNET SITES

Internet searchers must remember the importance of applying specific criteria to evaluate the reliability of a site. Who is providing the information? Where are the authors located? What is the currency of the information? Does the information offered have any research to back it up, and if so, is it cited? If you cannot find a site after previously visiting it, chances are it's a "fly-by-night" situation and therefore unreliable. One must be very certain of the information retrieved before following any of the recommendations it contains.

As Hwang pointed out recently:

> thousands of Web sites offer consumer health information and anyone with access and an interest can post health information on the Internet. Efforts are under way to assess quality health information on the Internet.[6]

Hwang suggests some ways of determining the validity of Internet health information, including the specific site's origin and funding, the frequency of the content's updating, the reviewers of the information and their credentials, and the sources of the information.[6]

Among the sites recommended by Hwang, OncoLink, sponsored by the University of Pennsylvania Medical Center and the University of Pennsylvania Cancer Center, provides comprehensive information about cancer and is located at <http://www.oncolink.upenn.edu>, and the Tufts University Nutrition Navigator, which provides links to nutrition information that has been reviewed by a team of nutrition experts, at <http://www.navigator.tufts.edu>, are outstanding.

Self-help and support groups raise many issues that should concern consumers. This topic continues to receive discussion in the literature as a concern for many in the medical field. Joan Stephenson recently noted that the "Internet as a medium is unusually conducive to deception."[7] She further cautions that those patients seeking medical information should remain highly alert to possible deception, particularly in online support groups. Some individuals are capable of pretense in order to gain attention.[7] Stephenson goes on to say that "The accessibility of online information makes it easy for people faking an illness to get details about their supposed condition."[7] However, this fact should not prevent consumers from investigating these methods for seeking information. Stephenson recommends that Internet users who seek patient information should remain aware of the possibility of victimization, but encourages them to take advantage of the positive benefits of support groups, including coping strategies and exchange of information about specific disease states.[7]

Newsgroups can help those consumers seeking others with the same or similar health conditions. Many newsgroups are available for this purpose. *Alt.health* and *Alt.med* are sites where users can discuss varieties of health and medical topics and issues. *Alt.support. cancer* provides an arena where users can discuss all types of cancers. *Alt.support.depression* offers a place for users to talk about depression and related issues. *Alt.support.epilepsy* gives a forum for discussion of epilepsy and seizures. One of the most important and popular newsgroups is *Go Ask Alice!* This question-and-answer service is from Columbia University Health Services. Users can submit questions or search a catalog of previous questions and answers on a variety of topics. The site is located at <http://www. columbia.edu/cu/healthwise/alice.html>. Those consumers wanting to discuss aspects on alternative health may find *misc.health. alternative* a useful newsgroup to visit. *Sci.med.aids* gives users a forum to discuss aspects of AIDS and HIV.

RECOMMENDED CONSUMER SITES ON THE INTERNET

Some specific sites deserve mention for consumers seeking health information on the Internet. An excellent site for patients seeking patient information on health-related topics such as headaches, sleep disorders, women's health, allergies, psychological disorders, infections, and addictions, only to suggest a few of the over 200 available subjects, is the American Academy of Family Physicians at <http://home.aafp.org/family/patient>. HealthWorld Online, at <http://www.healthy.net/>, presents a site divided into a variety of resources, including a Health Clinic, with articles on over 100 health conditions in a disease center, extensive information on women's and children's health, a cancer center, a natural medicine audio clinic, consumer laboratory services, and an alternative medicine center. The site emphasizes self-managed care, which appeals to many health consumers in today's world. The University of Kansas Medical Center provides a site with evaluated sources, available at <http://www.kumc.edu/service/dykes/dykeslib.html>. The biomedical Internet resources include a patient/consumer health information section, with topics such as allergy, cancer, chronic diseases, diabetes, and disabilities. Also noteworthy is the site The Internet Sleuth, at <http://www.isleuth.com/heal-index.html>, a database with directories of health sites using a single interface.

One of the very best health information sites comes from the Centers for Disease Control and Prevention, at <http://www.cdc.gov>. A wide variety of data is offered, including the full text of *Morbidity and Mortality Weekly Report (MMWR)*, many brochures, and access to CDC Wonder, a database with CDC reports, guidelines, and public health data, among many others. The Oregon Health Sciences University's site, at <http://www.ohsu.edu/cliniweb/>, provides quick and easy access to biomedical information on nearly 10,000 clinically oriented Web pages. This site also provides a link to the National Library of Medicine's PubMed database. The former Surgeon General, Dr. Koop, has a searchable site, at <http://www.drkoop.com/>, with many capabilities, among them a Virtual Pharmacy, Health Chat and Health Forums, a link to search both MEDLINE and CANCERLIT, health topics from allergies to travel health, health site reviews, and criteria for selection. It also has a resource center and many consumer-oriented items of information.

MedicineNet, a site operated by a group of board-certified physicians, has articles and links related to specific conditions and diseases. This site provides a question and answer service and searchable archive files with previous questions. Brief articles on prescription drugs, a medical dictionary, first aid information, and contacts to poison control centers are also available at <http://www.medicinenet.com>. MedMark, at <http://medmark.org/main.html>, offers medical resources listed by specialty, from anesthesiology to vascular surgery. Consumer health and patient education information is contained under each specialty topic. Links to many other sites are provided, including HealthAtoZ, at <http://www.healthatoz.com>, a database of thousands of sites in twenty-seven major subject areas.

The Michigan Electronic Library (MEL), at <http://mel.lib.mi.us/health/>, offers a site with multiple health information resources that have been selected and evaluated according to specific criteria. Considerable information on topics ranging from aging and alternative medicine/unconventional therapy to mental health, pain, and statistics is provided. ThriveOnline, at <http://www.thriveonline.com/community/thrive>, is a consumer health site with information on medicine, fitness, sports, diet, and sexuality. An extensive table of contents shows information available on topics such as AIDS/ HIV, alternative medicine, arthritis, asthma, back pain, cancer, and more.

Many associations offer sites on the World Wide Web, and several deserve mention as excellent resources for consumer health information. The American Association of Retired Persons, at <http://www. aarp.org/>, contains data and research on caregiving, healthy living, managed care, and rights of nursing home residents. The American Association for Geriatric Psychiatry, at <http://www.4woman.org/ nwhic/references/mdreferrals/aagp.htm>, is dedicated to promoting the mental health and well-being of older people and improving the care of those with late-life mental disorders. The mission of this organization focuses on enhancing the knowledge base and standard of practice in geriatric psychiatry through education and research, and it serves as an advocate for meeting the mental health needs of older Americans. The American Psychiatric Association, at <http:// www.psych.org/public_info/>, has as an organizational objective the advancement and improvement of care for persons with mental illnesses through nationwide public information, education, and awareness programs and materials. The site includes a consumer resources section with online versions of pamphlets on topics such as depression, coping with HIV/AIDS, Alzheimer's disease, eating disorders, and phobias. The American Social Health Association, at <http:// www.ashastd.org/>, has the mission to stop sexually transmitted diseases (STDs) and their harmful consequences to individuals, families, and communities. The site contains links to information and referral services, education and training, legislative advocacy, research, a National Herpes Hotline, a National AIDS Hotline, a National STD Hotline, and a National Immunization Information Hotline. The Arthritis Foundation, at <http://www.arthritis.org/>, has the mission of supporting research to find the cure for and prevention of arthritis. This site offers much valuable information, including a resource room containing educational brochures, fact sheets, lists of local services, and programs. A toll-free hotline for Arthritis Answers (1-800-283-7800) is provided, and a link to the "Fibromyalgia Wellness Letter" from the publishers of *Arthritis Today* makes this a particularly useful site.

The National Multiple Sclerosis Society, at <http://www.nmss.org/>, includes information and referral, programs for people who are newly diagnosed with MS, a lending library, a chapter newsletter, ongoing education programs, advocacy, and self-help groups. The society is dedicated to ending the devastating effects of MS and provides a toll-free number at 1-800-Fight-MS.

Many consumers find themselves searching for nontraditional methods of treating health problems. Chapter 7, "Alternative Medicine on the Net," provides much information on this topic. However, one particular site is well worth mentioning in this chapter. The National Institutes of Health's National Center for Complementary and Alternative Medicine, at <http://nccam.nih.gov>, sponsors a site from the office that facilitates research and evaluation of unconventional medical practices and disseminates this information to the public. A clearinghouse that serves as the public's point of contact and access to information makes the site a valuable one for consumers. The site also disseminates free fact sheets and provides information packages and publications about complementary and alternative medicine research supported by the National Institutes of Health. The toll-free number is 1-888-644-6226.

CONCLUSION

This chapter only touches the surface of options for consumers seeking health information from World Wide Web sites on the Internet. Readers should remember that the nature of the Internet is as a dynamic, fluid entity. Uniform resource locators (URLs) change frequently, and what was available at a specific site one day may not be there the next day. Because of this aspect, it will benefit the user to check on a site with some measure of regularity to make certain the information is being maintained at current levels.

REFERENCE NOTES

1. Eysenbach, G., and Diepgen, T.L. "Responses to Unsolicited Patient E-mail Requests for Medical Advice on the World Wide Web." *Journal of the American Medical Association* 280(October 21, 1998):1333-5.

2. Rose, S.; Bruce, J.; and Mafuli, N. "Accessing the Internet for Patient Information About Orthopedics." *Journal of the American Medical Association* 280(October 21, 1998):1309.

3. Lindberg, D.A.B., and Humphreys, B.L. "Medicine and Health on the Internet: The Good, the Bad, and the Ugly." *Journal of the American Medical Association* 280(October 21, 1998):1303-4.

4. Eng, T.R.; Maxfield, A.; Patrick, K. et al. "Access to Health Information and Support: A Public Highway or a Private Road?" *Journal of the American Medical Association* 280(October 21, 1998):1371-5.

5. "The Global Burden of Disease," World Health Organization World Bank, Lily Center for Women's Health, 1996, pp. 1-43.

6. Hwang, M.Y. "How to Find Reliable Online Health Information and Resources." *Journal of the American Medical Association* 280(October 21, 1998):1380.

7. Stephenson, J. "Patient Pretenders Weave Tangled 'Web' of Deceit." *Journal of the American Medical Association* 280(October 21, 1998):1297.

Chapter 7

Alternative Medicine on the Net

Suzanne M. Shultz
Nancy I. Henry
Esther Y. Dell

Alternative medicine is generally defined as therapy outside the scope of mainstream medical practice. It has also been described as complementary, integrated, or unconventional medicine. Whether one believes in the utility or efficacy of alternative medicine, about one-third of respondents to a survey published in the *New England Journal of Medicine* reported using an alternative therapy during the preceding year.[1] Alternatives are often used in conjunction with, intermittently with, or in place of conventional medicine. "Use" can range from an occasional supplement to an all-encompassing belief in a medical practice. The National Institute of Health's (NIH) National Center for Complementary and Alternative Medicine (NCCAM) has produced a broad classification of alternative medical practices: Mind-Body Medicine, Alternative Medical Systems, Lifestyle and Disease Prevention, Biologically Based Therapies, Manipulative and Body-Based Systems, Biofield, and Bioelectromagnetics. NCCAM says its list is neither complete nor authoritative (http://nccam.nih.gov/nccam/what-is-cam/classify.shtml).

People employ alternatives for a variety of reasons, but most commonly for treatment of a chronic or incurable disease or condition. Alternatives offer hope when other methods of treatment fail. Whereas physicians require scientifically valid evidence of effectiveness through controlled clinical trials and randomized controlled studies, alternative practitioners advocate the use of other criteria. Frequently, anecdotal accounts are all that support an alternative therapy.

If proof of effectiveness is difficult to establish by traditional methods, the problem is magnified manyfold on the Internet. The traditional screening process applied by publishers, either peer review or other measurable parameters, is often lacking on the Internet because everyone is potentially an individual writer/publisher. Anyone can alter, add, or delete information on the Internet. Traditional safeguards disappear, and an individual must independently assess the vast quantity of material available electronically.

Finding information about alternative medicine may prove relatively easy if health beliefs are cultural and one belongs to a particular cultural group. It is often common practice for families and friends to share complementary therapies from one generation to the next. Avenues of access would be known by relatives and friends and complementary therapies would be passed in the traditional sense, from person to person. For others, assimilation into American society frequently distances individuals from their cultural heritage. The global community of the Internet may prove instrumental in reconnecting individuals to their cultural ties and the wealth of information available related to complementary therapies.

KINDS OF ELECTRONIC
ALTERNATIVE HEALTH RESOURCES

There are as many kinds of electronic alternative health resources as there are print varieties. These include scholarly/informational, pamphlets and other technical reports, promotions/advertising, advocacy (attempts to influence opinion), news, organizations, and pharmaceutical resources. Not entirely unique to the electronic forum, although much more prevalent, is individual publishing. In this chapter, each of these categories will be defined and illustrated.

Scholarly or Informational Resources

Alternative medicine scholarly materials or information resources available on the Internet are those which meet the traditional tests of evaluation—author/authority, accuracy, objectivity, currency, and content—and are peer reviewed. Many are electronic format articles from reputable print-copy publications, such as the *Annals of Internal Medicine* or the *British Medical Journal*. These resources frequently reside in fee-for-service databases where full-text delivery is an option. Examples include Campion, "Why Unconventional Medicine?" from *New England Journal of Medicine*,[2] and Ullman, "The Mainstreaming of Alternative Medicine" from *Healthcare Forum*.[3] Both of these full-text papers may be viewed electronically for a fee through Ovid Technologies Full-Text option (http://www.ovid.com).

Scholarly journal excerpts or full-text papers are also available at no cost. For example, a randomized trial, "A Placebo-Controlled, Double Blind, Randomized Trial of an Extract of Gingko Biloba for Dementia" by Le Bars, P. L. and colleagues, was published in *JAMA (Journal of the American Medical Association)*.[4] This abstracted paper appears as a part of POEMS (Patient Oriented Evidence that Matters)—formerly JFP Journal Club—at the *Journal of Family Practice* Web site (http://www.infopoems.com). The entire paper may be found at the American Medical Association's scientific publications Web site, where selected full-text topics are available electronically (http://www. ama-assn.org/sci-pubs/journals/archive/jama/vol_278/no_16/71278. htm).

Individual Publishing

One advantage of the Internet is that it affords individuals and groups the ability to "publish" information much more easily than was previously possible. Self-publishing allows the author to control various aspects of the process, including editing, artwork, style, and so forth. However, individual publishing on the Internet suffers from the same drawback as its print counterpart, vanity publishing; that is, it escapes the peer-review process. Materials produced in this fashion are not necessarily without merit. "Basic Genetics: Cat Colours with Red" (http://freeusers.digibel.be/~crusade/genetics. htm) has more information on red cat genetics than the average browser could think to inquire about, but wisdom gleaned from this site will have little effect on the reader's health. Alternative medicine individual publishing is often of a promotional nature, such as "Treating Your Chronic Unwellness" by Dr. Joseph Mercola, in which certain dietary alterations and supplements are advocated (http://alternativehealthmall.com/info/herbsart.html).

Pamphlets and Pamphletlike Literature

Pamphlets have become the mainstay for specific or targeted information from specialty organizations, such as the American Heart Association, and for patient/consumer health information from hospitals, physicians, clinics, and health insurers. Desktop publishing has contributed to rapid expansion of pamphleteering as a means of information dissemination. Pamphlet-type literature on the Internet has also increased in volume and access. A pamphlet example is "What Is Naturopathic Medicine?" A free, brief, informational discourse on the philosophy and practice of natural medicine (http://www.pandamedicine.com/natmed.html), it would be typical of paper-copy pamphlet literature. An example of an electronic brochure is the American Holistic Veterinary Medical Association's "What Is Holistic Veterinary Medicine?" It describes various therapeutic options for animals, including chiropractic veterinary medicine, behavior modification, acupuncture, and meganutrients. Information on how to contact the association as well as a link to member practitioners, a description of the *Journal of the American Holistic Veterinary Medical Association*, annual meeting specifics, and education services may all be found at the Web site (http://www.altvetmed.com/AHVMA_brochure.html).

Promotion or Advertising

Much of the Internet is promotional, and it is important to differentiate between advertising and educational Web sites. The URL (uniform resource locator) provides the first clue about what to expect, for example, .com for commercial sites or .edu for educational ones. Alternative medicine product Web sites are limited only by the imagination and creativity of their owners/operators. A plethora of products is readily searchable. Alt-*MEDMarket* (http://alt.medmarket.com) calls itself your Internet source for alternative health products and services. There are numerous links to herbal, nutritional, and electromedical products (to name a few); the page is sponsored by a manufacturer of health and beauty products.

The Internet furnishes the means for purchase of alternative medicine products and services. Pycnogenol promotions extol the benefits of "a powerful antioxidant nutrient" that has been "in use since 1853" (http://seniorcosmetics.com/pycnogen.htm), and comes complete with a secure server allowing the use of a credit card for ordering. "Bioenergy Balancing with Marja West" (http://www.gems4friends.com/marja-west/) touts the healing potential of balancing the body's bioenergy fields and includes an address and phone number for appointments, information on workshops, and demonstrations.

Advocacy and Attempts to Influence Opinion

Closely linked to, and sometimes barely distinguishable from, advertising, advocacy defends, pleads, or supports an idea, product, behavior, or therapy. For alternative medicine sites, advocacy may take the form of anecdotal or discursive product promotions. "Multiple Sclerosis: A New, Non-Drug, Natural Approach" is an example of a testimonial that includes personal experiences, a form to request a complimentary tape, an audio clip from an expert in support of the product, and thirty-two references (http://www.naturalresource.com/multiple.html). Other testimonials can be found through links at the same site.

A grandiloquent product promotion is exemplified by "Defender; the highest quality grape seed extract antioxidant available today!" at Ideal Solutions Web site (http://www.netside.net/~c3i/defender.html). Here again, one may request a cassette tape that explains the benefits of the product. A handy cost-per-unit price comparison with similar products extols the low cost and superior quality of "Defender," manufactured and distributed by Ideal Solutions International—synergistic products designed to assist the body int he natural processes of weight loss, hormone balance, free radical control, and general health and well-being.

News

Many of the health and medicine Web sites offer a service, link, or subsection that reports the latest medical news, sometimes on a daily basis. A well-known news service is Reutershealth, which offers a professional (by subscription) news service and a consumer (free) health eLine service (http://www.reutershealth.com).

Samples of alternative medicine news pages are those linked to NOAH (New York Online Access to Health) (http://www.noah.cuny.edu/alternative/alternative.html#Online); *Healthy Update*, a Health-world Online publication; and *Wellness Newsletter*, from Wellspring Media. *Wellness Newsletter*, with available back issues, covers such timely topics as chakras, fen-phen, and kombucha tea. *Healthy Update* profiled a recent *Journal of the American Medical Association* publication and reviewed trends in the U.S. vitamin industry.

Alternative Healthcare and Wellness is a daily news page from NewsEdge corporation providing a few relevant alternative therapy stories of several paragraphs each (http://www.newspage.com/browse/46610/46611/283).

Organizations

With each passing day, more organizations provide information about themselves on the Internet. Information about numerous alternative medicine organizations and foundations, which vary from the eminently respectable to the questionable, populates the Web. Some examples include (1) the American Association of Naturopathic Physicians, a busy, colorful site (http://www.Naturopathic.org/Welcome.html); (2) Herb Research Foundation (Boulder, Colorado), a non-profit research and educational foundation that offers reliable herbal information (http://www.herbs.org); (3) NIH's National Center for Complementary and Alternative Medicine, created by Congress to evaluate and determine the effectiveness of alternative therapies (http://nccam.nih.gov/); and (4) the Association of Natural Medicine Pharmacists, dedicated to those seeking professional information and education. The association sponsors a clearinghouse for factual, not anecdotal, natural medicine (http://www.anmp.org).

Pharmaceutical Resources

Drug manufacturers and pharmaceutical information also abound on the Internet. Companies vary from such well-established corporations as the Eli Lilly Company to less well-known businesses, and the quality of presentation is highly variable. A few examples of alternative medicine pharmaceutical sites include Intelligent Choice, Incorporated (http://www.absolutelyhealthy.com/ishii/index.html), which claims to be "the world leading manufacturer of pristine quality nutritional supplements." The company's product line comes from Japan and is "market proven." This site has grammatical and spelling errors on the first page! The Nature's Answer Web site (http://www.bio-botanica.com), a division of Bio-Botanica, manufactures liquid herbal extracts. The home page contains the company's mission and a statement on commitment to herbal research and adherence to quality control standards in herbal extract manufacturing. The latest Web page revision date is posted in the footer. Other pages at the site (1) detail herbal extract products and ordering information, (2) present a directory, glossary, and quick reference guide of herbal names and uses, and (3) list mail, telephone, and e-mail contacts for the company. Olympian Labs, Incorporated, "creators of the finest nutritional supplements," produces anti-oxidants, vitamins, minerals, and herbal products (http://www. Olympian-Labs.com/). The opening product page contains an anecdotal account in support of one of the company's creations. There are detailed merchandise descriptions, including order numbers and quantities by which the products are sold, but no prices. Contact information (phone, fax, and mail) is provided as well as the Webmaster's e-mail.

Bibliographic Databases

A number of premium (fee-based) databases specialize or focus on alternative medicine and natural therapies and can be accessed via the Internet. Among these are (1) AMED—Allied and Alternative Medicine—produced by the British Library and available from DataStar/Dialog, covering fields of complementary or alternative medicine from 1985 to the present (http://ds.datastarweb.com/ds/products/datastar/sheets/amed.htm); (2) EMED-EMBASE—produced by Elsevier and available from DataStar/Dialog, covering pharmacology and related medicine since 1974 (http://ds.datastarweb.com/ds/products/datastar/sheets/emed.htm); (3) MANT—Manual, Alternative and Natural Therapy MANTIS—produced by Action Potential and available from DataStar/Dialog, covering chiropractic and osteopathic medicine from 1880 forward and alternative medicine from 1990 to the present (http://ds.datastarweb.com/ds/products/datastar/sheets/mant.htm); (4) IBIS—Interactive Body Mind Information System—produced by Integrative Medical Arts Group, covering natural medicine/therapeutics and complementary health care (http://www.integrative-medicine.com) (IBIS is not truly a database, but a full-text resource on diseases and therapeutics); and (5) NAPRALERT, the Natural Products Alert File (http://info.cas.org/ONLINE/catalog/napralert.html), produced by the University of Illinois College of Pharmacy. NAPRALERT is a fee-for-service, bibliographic, and factual database on natural products from 1650 to the present.

Free databases may be found in PubMed (http://www.ncbi.nlm.nih.gov/ PubMed), the National Library of Medicine's bibliographic database offering 9 million records from 1966 to the present, and CAM Citation Index from the National Center for Complementary and Alternative Medicine (http://nccam.nih.gov/ncresources/cam-ci/), a searchable database of 90,000 records extracted from MEDLINE from 1966 to 1997. Alternative medicine databases are covered in greater detail by Snow in *Database*, June/July 1998.[5]

Strauss commented on the quality of medical information on the Internet, noting, "Clearly, medical pages on the Internet are a mixed bag. Some sites are excellent and others are just plain scary; nonetheless all are equally accessible online."[6] The quality of alternative medicine pharmaceutical sites is very uneven and should be viewed critically, applying as many evaluative techniques as possible.

Finding information on the Internet does not seem to be the challenge, but rather identifying the carefully researched information relevant to your particular question.

Search Engines

There seems to be no limit to the abundance of free information available on the Internet. The lack of command language and controlled vocabulary is particularly unnerving to knowledgeable librarians and other professional searchers. If two words are entered on the search screen, the engine matches all words giving hits with both words first, assuming that they are the most relevant. For example, search terms *alternative medicine* yield 1,131,521 hits in Excite and 10,439,050 in AltaVista. The list of results provides a brief description of the best matches in descending order, with the most relevant first. Fortunately, related or similar Web sites tend to link to one another, so even an inexact search strategy may yield a relevant result. Additional techniques may be suggested by a help menu called "search tips" at the individual search engine sites, providing examples of how to limit by time frames, Boolean operators, language, filtering "out" words, searching only the first or top page at each Web site, or expanding by using wild cards (*) to truncate words, paying attention to case sensitivities (lowercase usually yields more) and using the "more like this" options.

A search engine review chart was used to determine the most powerful search engines currently available to retrieve information on the World Wide Web (http://searchenginewatch.com/reports/reviewchart.html). Using the selected search engines, a comparative chart was formulated to report the results. Since alternative medicine commonly goes by other descriptors, terms used to execute these searches included "alternative medicine," "integrated medicine," "complementary medicine," "unorthodox medicine," and "unconventional medicine." Quotation marks around each search strategy were used to indicate that the words should be considered as a phrase and not individually. Using quotes reduced hits in Excite to 22,210 and in AltaVista to 52,582. Table 7.1 summarizes the results.

Links

Many Web sites on the Internet point to, or link with, sites similar to their own. Using these electronic reference sources can help to locate additional relevant information or expand upon a special interest.

The University of Pittsburgh's Alternative Medicine home page (http://www.pitt.edu/~cbw/altm.html) refers the user to other Internet resources on alternative therapies. The "Databases" link includes some unique entries. The page, when last visited, had been updated within the last three months.

CAMPS (Complementary and Alternative Medicine Program at Stanford), sponsored by the Stanford Center for Research and Disease Prevention (http://scrdp.stanford.edu/camps.html), includes a resources page for reference. It does not endorse any of the groups listed. Neither the creators nor the last update were apparent.

TABLE 7.1. Search Engine Comparison (October 6, 1998)

	HOT BOT	INFO SEEK	EXCITE	ALTA-VISTA	YAHOO	LYCOS	WEB CRAWLER[a]
"alternative medicine"[b]	47,471	53,126	13,630	59,557	144	100	1,640
"integrated medicine"	585	275	223	601	5	100	28
"complementary medicine"	6,619	3,848	5,970	9,325	26	100	212
"unorthodox medicine"	60	38	14	88	14	100	0
"unconventional medicine"	383	197	137	544	160	100	17

a Search engines in rank order 1 through 7 derived from <http://searchenginewatch.com/reports/reviewchart.html>.
b Search strategy, in quotations (except Lycos).

Directories or Guides

A directory conjures up an image of a computer file or a telephone book. For our purposes, directories are classified lists that pertain to a specific subject. A number of alternative medicine directories on the Internet combine a number of Web site resources on alternative medicine topics.

MedWeb—Emory University Health Sciences Center Library (http://www.medweb.emory.edu/MedWeb/FmPro)—provides several pages of alphabetically arranged alternative medicine subjects from societies and associations to kombucha. Virtually all aspects of alternative therapy, including techniques, literature and resources, diseases, beliefs, conferences, and academic programs, may be found through links provided at this site. EINet Virtual Medical Library (http://galaxy.einet.net/galaxy/medicine/therapeutics/Alternative-Medicine.html) "Alternative Medicine" (subject) selection provides a comprehensive list of links to therapeutic options and references two additional directories. Dr. Bower's Complementary and Alternative Medicine home page (http://www.people.virginia.edu/~pjb3s/Complementary_Practices.html) is a comprehensive list of alternative and complementary medicine topics maintained by Peter J. Bower, MD. HealthWWWeb: Integrative Medicine, Natural Health and Alternative Therapies (http://www.healthwwweb.com/) includes Web resources, books, journals, a resource guide, a discussion group, health information tools, schools, and events. Healthfinder (http://www.healthfinder.org), a U.S. Department of Health and Human Services consumer health information gateway, presents a short directory to alternative medicine Web sites and organizations. Healthfinder claims to help "consumers find reliable health information from many Federal agencies, States, professional associations, nonprofit organizations and universities" so that "users don't have to surf the Net to find the links they want."[7]

Organizations often include directories to assist in locating alternative health practitioners at their Web sites. Examples include "Practitioners Directories" linked to the alternative medicine home page (http://www.pitt.edu/~cbw/pract.html); Alternative Health Practitioners from Natural Health Resources (http://healthy.photobbs.com/); or the

American Academy of Medical Acupuncture Referral Index (http://
www.medicalacupuncture.org/referral.htm).

Reviews

Ranking or review mechanisms are frequently marketed as a value-added service provided by individual search engines to select the "Best of the Web" or top Web sites. However, review criteria may be related to issues other than content, and the names or expertise of reviewers may not be apparent. For example, *Lycos Top 5% Best of the Web* is touted as a selective list of top-shelf sites that are rated by the Web's most experienced reviewers. The editorial staff at Lycos use excellence as their only rating criterion and they re-review the site only if significant changes occur. The rating categories are content (useful, accurate, and up to date), design (beautiful, colorful, and user friendly), and overall (fun, inviting, and captivating.) To clarify the rating scale, comparisons (0-100) are made with classic rock bands; the Beatles, Rolling Stones, and Bob Dylan types are in the top 90 to 100.

Education World's Education Site Reviews assigns ratings based on content, aesthetics, and organization; a short description of the high points of the site round out the "A" through "F" grade-rating review.

Webcrawler "Top Sites" for Alternative Medicine (http://
webcrawler.com/health/alternative_medicine/) includes a short list of five very popular sites and a somewhat longer list of "More Sites." No explanation for site selection accompanies the page so the criteria are unknown. Several of the Web sites in the secondary list (University of Pittsburgh's Alternative Medicine home page, MedWeb—Alternative Medicine from Emory University, and National Center for Complementary and Alternative Medicine) would be more appropriately assigned to the "Top" list based upon content and accuracy.

Newsgroups

Newsgroups are discussion groups organized by people with a similar interest. They function similar to a public e-mail system where all subscribers, and in some cases anyone, can read the postings. A sample of discussion groups for alternative medicine may be found at

HealthyWay Health Links News and Discussion Groups (http://www1. sympatico.ca/healthway/COMMUNITIES/alt_com.html). A substantial annotated list and a link to obtain instructions for subscribing to news-groups are packed onto a single page.

EVALUATION

Evaluation of information has traditionally been a function of the research librarian. There are six tried-and-true criteria upon which to base an evaluation: author, authority, accuracy, objectivity, currency, and purpose. Electronic sources encompass an additional set of evaluative criteria of general (how does it look and feel?) and specific (what about links and fonts?) nature. Because the Internet is used on a more individual basis, that is, the information is not filtered by an intermediary such as an editorial board, the end user must ultimately determine the validity of the information.

Traditional bibliographic criteria apply to all scholarly Internet Web documents, not exclusively to alternative medicine sites. The *author* should be readily discernible and knowledgeable about the subject on which he/she is writing. For this reason, biographical information and credibility are important. Education and credentials help to determine reliability but are not guarantees of *authority*. The user must determine if there is bias in the author's presentation and whether the credentials are accurate and respected. Is the author affiliated with an organization, a company, or an educational institution?

True *objectivity* is difficult to achieve. Organizations usually exist for a purpose; authors may write for reasons other than scientific contribution. In evaluating a Web document, one should look for information that is balanced and as free of bias as possible. Check for obvious conflicts of interest. If the document is peer-reviewed, check the reviewers or the responsible organizations for their reputation in the discipline. Goals should be apparent; is this essay advertising or informational? Facts should be clearly stated, with no inconsistencies or contradictions; documents should be free of spelling and grammatical errors.

The material presented should, ideally, be evidence based, reproducible, and verifiable. A search of the Cochrane Database of Systematic Reviews yielded only eight citations indexed to alternative medicine, while a search of PubMed using the "Advanced Search" option indexed to the MeSH headings "alternative medicine" and "randomized controlled trials" produced ninety-eight citations. These quality filtering devices and systems do not apply universally to the scientific medical literature, nor are they (or similar tools) yet available for the majority of sites on the Internet.

Currency is a major advantage of the Internet over other information sources; documentation of the original "publication" date and the last update should be easily discernible. While it is readily accepted that print documents may be months or years old, Web documents are expected to be current within days or weeks.

Silberg believes that medical sources on the Internet must, at a minimum, meet the standards of authorship (credentials), attribution (references and sources), disclosure (ownership/sponsorship), and currency (dates posted/updated).[8] In addition, *purpose, scope,* and *coverage* should be considered. The reader should be able to determine whether the piece exists to inform or to persuade. Scope and coverage entail examination of the information for range (balanced picture), accuracy (factual), and audience. Are all the facts available, and are there any omissions? Internet alternative medicine sites and documents should be compared with print and other formats of similar information and checked for references. This confirmation process helps determine validity and is recognized as integral to the scientific research process.

While the traditional evaluation of an Internet Web site is a critical first test, there are a number of electronic-specific criteria that are equally important. First, and probably most significant, is ease of location. The site or document must be accessible from a known search engine by simple word association or by link from a site found by a search engine. A site that is arcane is the same as a reference that cannot be located. Once found and recorded, the Web site must be stable; that is, it must be there the next time one goes back to it or, at least, provide a viable forwarding address.

Ideally, a document should include standard Web anatomy. Standard Web anatomy includes a header that clearly states its topic or title, a body of information, and a footer with date, revision date, and sponsor. Author, compiler, or Webmaster information should appear in either the header or footer.

A Web document should be readable and usable. The use of fonts, graphics, and animation may add interest but should not obscure the message.

Links from the home or main page facilitate usability and may function similar to an outline or index at the Web site. Selection criteria and link annotations help to clarify the reasons for addenda to the site. These features indicate that the page was well thought out. If the site is very large, an internal search function would provide ease of navigation.

A journal article in *Lancet* critiqued the practice of framing in Web sources.[9] Framing is a method of presenting information on a page using tables and so forth, from a noncommercial source, wrapping it in commercial advertising material, and showing the aggregate as a whole package. Framing blurs the line between types of information sources; commercial entities include research materials to increase the status of their products. The advertisement draws on the credibility of the original source. This practice makes information even more difficult to validate because "selected information" may be taken out of context to prove a point. Each individual part of a Web site should be evaluated for quality and the entire document for internal consistency and validity.

Medical Advice on the Net

The Geneva-based Health On the Net Foundation publishes a code of conduct for medical and health Web sites that is embodied in eight principles (http://www.hon.ch/HONcode/Conduct.html). They are as follows:

1. Medical advice at this Web site is offered only by qualified medical professionals.
2. Information is designed to support the physician-patient relationship.
3. Patients/visitors to the Web site can expect privacy to be respected.
4. Information given will be supported by references.
5. Claims made will be supported by evidence.

6. Information will be clear and contacts' addresses provided; Webmaster will be published.
7. Any commercial or noncommercial support of the Web site will be identified.
8. If advertising is a source of funding, it will be identified.

These tenets address quality of content and provide some assurance that the information displayed is reliable.

Two studies that appeared during the last year uncovered less than adequate net coverage of two common childhood conditions, according to comment or article: fever in the *British Medical Journal*, June 1997,[10] and diarrhea in *Pediatrics*, June 1998.[11] As more studies such as these are conducted, it is to be hoped that Web pages will be motivated to provide better, more reliable information.

ALTERNATIVE MEDICINE RESEARCH OPPORTUNITIES

Research trials on alternative therapies are being conducted worldwide. In MEDLINE, the preponderance of centers involved in investigation are European and Canadian, with a few isolated hospitals and universities in the United States conducting single randomized controlled trials. Nuffield Department of Anaesthetics, University of Oxford, the Churchill, England; the Research Council for Complementary Medicine, London, United Kingdom; Centre for Complementary Medical Research, Technische Universität/Ludwig-Maximillians-Universität, Munich, Germany; Department of Complementary Medicine, Postgraduate Medical School, University of Exeter, United Kingdom; Institute for Research in Extramural Medicine, Vrije Universität, Amsterdam, Netherlands; and various departments at McMaster University, Hamilton, Ontario, Canada, have conducted more than one randomized controlled trial of an alternative therapy. In addition, the Cochrane Collaboration produced eight research projects in 1998 that were indexed to alternative medicine. The National Center for Complementary and Alternative Medicine (http://nccam.nih.gov/nccam/) lists eleven centers in the United States that are currently conducting research in areas ranging from addictions to women's health issues.

SUMMARY

It is important to note that although the Internet provides rapid access to an abundance of information resources on alternative medicine/complementary practices, the reliability of these sources requires validation. For many users, the need to validate resources may be a foreign concept, and even for those who understand the necessity of the validation process, applying the necessary criteria may prove too cumbersome. For this reason, librarians familiar with research and evaluation processes may be the most valuable initial contact for persons attempting to locate this type of information. The general user does not understand the difference between the kind of information found in a research library versus a public library, that is, that the information is already evaluated through the collection development process. Methods to evaluate alternative medicine sources and efficacy of alternative therapies are still in their infancy. As research methodology improves, it will translate into more reliable literature resources in "print" and on the "Net." The controversies still make this a difficult process, not entirely dissimilar to conventional treatment options where *only* the patient can ultimately determine therapeutic usefulness.

REFERENCE NOTES

1.   Eisenberg, D.M.; Kessler, R.C.; Foster, C. et al. "Unconventional Medicine in the United States. Prevalence, Costs and Patterns of Use." *New England Journal of Medicine* 328(January 28, 1993):246-252.

2.   Campion, E.W. "Why Unconventional Medicine?" *New England Journal of Medicine* 328(January 28, 1993):282-23.

3.   Ullman, D. "The Mainstreaming of Alternative Medicine." *Healthcare Forum* 36 (November/December 1993):24-30.

4.   Le Bars, P.L.; Katz, M.M.; Berman. N. et al. "A Placebo-Controlled, Double-blind, Randomized Trial of an Extract of Ginkgo Biloba for Dementia. North American EGb Study Group." *JAMA* 278(October 22, 1997):1327-32.

5.   Snow, B. "Alternative Medicine; Information Sources." *Database* 21(June/July 1998):19-29.

6.   Strauss, K. "Quality of Medical Information on the Internet." *JAMA* 278(August 27, 1997):632.

7.   Healthfinder: A Gateway to Online Consumer Health Information Produced by the Federal Government and Its Many Partners. Pamphlet. April 21, 1998.

8.   Silberg, W.M.; Lundberg, G.D.; and Musacchio, R.A. "Assessing, Controlling, and Assuring the Quality of Medical Information on the Internet: Caveant Lector et Viewor—Let the Reader and Viewer Beware." *JAMA* 277(April 16, 1997):1244-5.

9.   "The Web of Information Inequality." *Lancet* 349(June 21, 1997):1781.

10.   Impicciatore, P.; Pandolfini, C.; Casella, N.; et al. "Reliability of Health Information for the Public on the World Wide Web; Systematic Survey of Advice on Managing Fever in Children at Home." *BMJ* 314 (June 28, 1997):1875-9.

11.   McClung, H.J.; Murray, R.D.; and Heitlinger, L.A. "The Internet As a Source for Current Patient Information." *Pediatrics* 101(June 1, 1998):E2.

Chapter 8

Government Resources on the Net

Nancy J. Allee

Good information is the best medicine. Immediate access to current medical research information is as critical as the biopsy and the x-ray have been in the diagnosis and treatment of disease. Not only health professionals, but also consumers, should have the most recent medical information at their fingertips.[1]

Michael E. DeBakey, MD

INTRODUCTION

This chapter is written for a diverse audience encompassing both experienced and novice searchers, that is, an audience that may include reference librarians who, although knowledgeable about Internet resources in general, would find useful an introductory guide to specific government resources in the area of health information, as well as individuals and health care consumers who may be new to searching the Internet and have an interest in locating government resources available electronically.

Even though a vast amount of health-related government information is available through the Internet and accessible via Telnet, Gopher,

This chapter was completed with the valued assistance of colleagues at the University of Michigan: Barbara Hegenbart, Matt Krupa, Helen Look, Melissa McCollum, Janelle Neroda, Michele Saunders, Anna Schnitzer, Ayke Tjandra, and Linda Whang. Special appreciation and gratitude is extended to Grace York for reviewing chapter content.

FTP (file transfer protocol), and other methods, the scope of this chapter is focused on those resources which are accessible through the World Wide Web, hereafter referred to as the Web, and on those resources pertaining to international, federal, and state government information, with particular emphasis on U.S. government resources. Government information is statistically intensive; therefore, this chapter will highlight some of the major Internet sites containing health statistics. Readers are also recommended to consult Chapter 9, "Health-Related Statistical Information on the Net," for more comprehensive coverage of this topic. Content of this chapter will be a combination of annotated government sites providing health-related information and techniques and strategies for accessing them.

POINTS OF ACCESS

The number of current Web sites continues to increase at a dramatic pace, with estimates ranging from 60 to 100 million pages, a number that appears to double at four-month intervals.[2] Government resources alone, identified by .gov (government) and .mil (military) domain name extensions, are estimated to comprise over 1 million sites.[3] Government sites are proliferating for a variety of reasons, two of which can be traced to outcomes of the Paperwork Reduction Act of 1980 (http://www.whitehouse.gov/WH/EOP/OMB/html/circulars/a130/a130.html), aimed at reducing the regulatory burden of disseminating government information, and the Government Printing Office Electronic Information Access Enhancement Act of 1993, known as the "GPO Access Law," requiring GPO to make government publications available electronically with free access provided to depository libraries.[4,5]

The increasing number of Web sites and their impermanent nature as the Web presently exists creates a challenge for information specialists and consumers to locate and evaluate reliable sources that will endure and remain available for future consultation and other archival purposes. One proposed solution to the ever-changing Web is implementation of permanent identifiers to replace the current system of temporal Web addresses using the uniform resource locator (URL) mechanism for linking pages.[6] In fact, the Federal Depository Library Program has recently announced that PURLs (permanent uniform resource locators) have been implemented into the GPO Pathway Service for providing continued bibliographic access to government Internet resources.[7] Another solution to successful Web searching in terms of locating reliable sites is to consult directories focused on the specific type and content of the subject information one is seeking, thereby maximizing both time and results.[6] The following information is designed to link users to government health information utilizing the most direct methods of access.

TRADITIONAL SOURCES

Several standard texts are helpful in providing overviews to government resources; among these are Joe Morehead's *Introduction to United States Government Information Sources*[8] and Roper and Boorkman's *Introduction to Reference Sources in the Health Sciences,*[9] which includes a chapter on government publications. Additionally, there are texts that focus on electronic government resources, among which are Judith Robinson's *Tapping the Government Grapevine: The User-Friendly Guide to U.S. Government Information Sources,*[5] John Maxymuk's *Finding Government Information on the Internet,*[4] Bruce Maxwell's *How to Access the Federal Government on the Internet*[10] and *How to Find Health Information on the Internet,*[11] Greg Notess's *Government Information on the Internet,*[3] and the *1998 Guide to Health Care Resources on the Internet,* edited by John Hoben.[12]

To elaborate on those texts that focus specifically on electronic information, *Tapping the Government Grapevine* is in its third edition and continues to be an exceptional resource for demystifying government information resources and bibliographic access to them in a user-friendly fashion, as indicated by the book's subtitle and by examples of the author's metaphor-infused commentary on the changing nature and challenge of locating information on the Web: "Describing Web sites is like narrating action at a bird feeder. Flux is frequent and without fanfare" and "The quest for government information can make even seasoned library users and senior librarians cringe like vampires recoiling from sunlight."[5] Robinson's book contains substantial new Internet material and covers the depository library system; the history and purpose of the Government Printing

Office (GPO); search techniques for a variety of electronic resources, including the Library of Congress's THOMAS database and MOCAT, the *Monthly Catalog of United States Government Publications*, a comprehensive index of both depository and nondepository publications and both GPO and non-GPO materials; and scientific, legislative, executive, and judicial Internet information resources. The chapter on scientific resources is particularly useful in identifying Internet health resources.

Similar to Robinson's book, Maxymuk's *Finding Government Information on the Internet* provides helpful background information on the Government Printing Office and the Depository Library Program and poses significant questions about the future roles and responsibility of each in the context of the dissemination of government information in the age of electronic resource delivery. The book includes a chapter titled "Health, Medicine, and the Environment," providing a brief overview of selected government sites relevant to these topics.

Maxwell's *How to Access the Federal Government on the Internet* features descriptions of over 400 Internet sites, including not only Web pages but also Gopher, FTP, and Telnet sites, in addition to e-mail groups on particular topics. The same author also publishes *How to Find Health Information on the Internet*, an extensive subject guide to a wide variety of electronic resources, including government Web sites.

Notess's *Government Information on the Internet* is a well-organized, well-researched, evaluative listing of over 1,200 federal, state, and international government Internet resources that includes a chapter on health-related information.

The *1998 Guide to Health Care Resources on the Internet* contains ten chapters addressing various issues surrounding Internet technology and health information, with government sites interspersed with commercial and educational Web resources. Particularly noteworthy are chapters covering pharmaceutical information and consumer health information. The book also includes a section evaluating the "Top 25" Web sites in the areas of health policy, managed care, outcomes research, home care resources, ambulatory resources, disease management, quality management, and electronic data interchange, several of which are government sites.

Sears and Moody[13] have identified a five-category approach to developing a search strategy for government information, including known item (e.g., title), agency, subject, statistics, and special techniques. Hersh concurs that "Information sources, print or computer, are approached for two reasons: the need to locate a particular item of information . . . or the need to obtain information on a particular subject."[14] Sears and Moody's approach, although developed for print-based resources, has applications in an electronic environment. It, along with Hersh's emphasis on locating particular items and subject-specific searches, will be adopted as a guiding framework for discussing access to Web-based government resources.

WEB SOURCES

This approach employs the Internet itself, rather than standard print sources such as bibliographies, guides, and directories, as the starting point for locating government sites.

Known Item/Title Searches

As mentioned earlier, more and more government resources, formerly available only in print, are now accessible via the Web. When searching for a specific item or publication's availability on the Internet, one might begin by using one of the many commercial search engines available on the Web (AltaVista at <http://www.altavista.com/>, Excite at <http://www.excite.com/>, InfoSeek at <http://guide.infoseek.com/>, Lycos at <http://www.lycos.com/>, or Yahoo! at <http://www.yahoo.com/>, among others) and simply enter the title of the publication, such as *Healthy People 2000 Review* or *Statistical Abstract of the United States* or *Health, United States* or *The United States Government Manual,* to name a few of the general and health-related government publications now available on the Internet. In terms of search strategy and maximizing retrieval relevancy and efficiency, note the search options or search help screens for each search engine that explain the mechanics of search retrieval within that site. For instance, retrieval by publication title is more efficient at Yahoo!'s site when the option *"exact phrase match"* is selected and more efficient at AltaVista when, for example, a search for the title *Health, United States* is entered as *"health, united states"* (quotation marks inclusive). The various search engine sites can also be used to locate specific government entities by simply entering the name of the organization or service unit, such as the National Technical Information Service or the Government Printing Office.

In addition to commercial sites, however, there are several recommended Web resources within the government itself that are available for identifying and locating health information. The following annotated list of Web sites is a selective guide to government health information categorized by title, agency, subject, statistical sources, and special interest sites. Highlights of health-related information are noted, but readers are encouraged to explore in depth the Web pages at each site for more comprehensive information.

Catalog of United States Government Publications (MOCAT)
<http://www.access.gpo.gov/su_docs/dpos/adpos400.html>

An online catalog to information resources available through the Federal Depository Library Program. The bibliographic data are updated daily and are searchable by title (fielded search), keyword, agency, report number, Superintendent of Documents class number, depository number, and Government Printing Office sales stock number.

Uncle Sam Migrating Government Publications
<http://www.lib.memphis.edu/gpo/mig.htm>

This site, maintained by the Regional Depository Library of the University of Memphis, provides an A to Z title listing of links to government publications that are available in full-text electronic format.

Agency Searches

How many government agencies are in existence? Currently, the number is approximately 5,800,[5] which reinforces the importance of mechanisms for effective retrieval. This section first identifies

Internet resources that are helpful search tools for locating government agencies and government Web sites by subject, then focuses on those agencies which fall under the aegis of the Department of Health and Human Services (DHHS), a premier resource for government health information. It also makes note of other agencies and government organizations related to health care at the federal, state, and international levels.

Federal Web Locator
<http://www.law.vill.edu/fed-agency/fedwebloc.html>

This site is maintained by the Center for Information Law and Policy, a joint initiative of the Illinois Institute of Technology's Chicago-Kent College of Law and the Villanova University School of Law; it features searching capability by federal agency name.

U.S. Federal Government Agencies Directory
<http://www.lib.lsu.edu/gov/fedgov.html>

This site is maintained by Louisiana State University and provides links to federal government agencies represented in the *United States Government Manual.*

Subject Searches

FEDWORLD
<http://www.fedworld.gov/#usgovt>

This site, established by the National Technical Information Service (NTIS), serves as a directory to federal government and business information and features keyword searching via the following: the FEDWORLD Information Network, U.S. Government Reports, and U.S. Government Web Sites.

GovBot
<http://ciir2.cs.umass.edu/Govbot/>

Developed by the Center for Intelligent Information Retrieval, this site provides keyword searching of over 1 million federal government and military Web resources.

GPO Browse Topics
<http://www.access.gpo.gov/su_docs/dpos/pathbrws.html>

This site, maintained by GPO Pathway Services, features A to Z links to government Internet sites.

GPO Monthly Catalog
<http://www.access.gpo.gov/su_docs/dpos/adpos400.html>

This is an online catalog to information resources available through the Federal Depository Library Program. The bibliographic data are updated daily and are searchable by title (fielded search), keyword, agency, report number, Superintendent of Documents class number, depository number, and Government Printing Office sales stock number.

GPO Pathway Services
<http://www.access.gpo.gov/su_docs/aces/aces760.html>

Described as a "suite of tools being continually developed by the Federal Depository Library Program to direct librarians and the public to Federal Government information on the Internet," this site provides links to the Government Information Locator Service (GILS), federal agency Internet sites, and searchable agency databases.

Federal Agencies, Department of Health and Human Services

Department of Health and Human Services (DHHS)
<http://www.os.dhhs.gov/>

This site provides links to the offices and agencies that comprise DHHS, as well as links to resources on federal grant programs, organ donation, and the health status of special populations such as adolescents. Especially noteworthy is Healthfinder (http://www.healthfinder. gov), a gateway to consumer health and human services information from the U.S. government, cosponsored by the Office of Disease Prevention and Health Promotion and the National Health Information Center. Healthfinder includes an A to Z subject guide for retrieving information on specific topics.

Agency for Health Care Policy and Research (AHCPR)
<http://www.ahcpr.gov/>

AHCPR's target audience is medical practitioners and consumers and other purchasers of health care services. The agency is comprised of eleven offices and centers with responsibility for conducting research and implementing programs to improve the quality of health care. The site provides links to consumer health information topics, such as smoking cessation and stroke prevention in addition to survey information, such as the Medical Expenditure Panel Survey on health care utilization, expenditures, and insurance coverage for defined populations. Information is also available in Spanish.

Agency for Toxic Substances and Disease Registry (ATSDR)
<http://atsdr1.atsdr.cdc.gov:8080/atsdrhome.html>

ATSDR provides health information in accordance with its mission to prevent exposure to, and assess the effects of, hazardous substances in the environment. The site includes national alerts on toxic substances, health advisories, reports on topics such as multiple chemical sensitivity, information about toxicological impacts of Superfund hazardous waste sites, and a list of the top twenty hazardous substances on the ATSDR/EPA (Environmental Protection Agency) Priority List. Also available at this site is HazDat, ATSDR's database for accessing substance interactions, effects of exposure to hazardous substances, and other health information pertaining to Superfund sites and impacts on populations and the environment.

Centers for Disease Control and Prevention (CDC)
<http://www.cdc.gov/>

The CDC is comprised of eleven offices and centers with responsibility for disease and injury prevention and control. The CDC's home page provides links to each of the individual centers, institutes, and offices, which include the National Center for Chronic Disease Prevention and Health Promotion; the National Center for Infectious Diseases; the National Institute for Occupational Safety and Health; the National Center for HIV, STD, and TB Prevention; and the Office of Women's Health. (The CDC's National Center for Health Statistics and CDC Wonder are discussed later in this chapter on pp. 146-147) Also available at the site are A-Z links to health information on topics ranging from asthma, arthritis, bicycle-related head injuries, cancer, ebola viral hemorrhagic fever, rabies, and spina bifida to yellow fever; an online version of the Global Health Odyssey, which details the history of public health in America and CDC's efforts to prevent disease and injury; and links to publications such as the peer-reviewed electronic journal *Emerging Infectious Diseases*, published by the National Center for Infectious Diseases, and *Morbidity and Mortality Weekly Review*.

Food & Drug Administration (FDA)
<http://www.fda.gov/default.htm>

The FDA ensures the safety of food, cosmetics, medicines, medical devices, and radiation-emitting products. The site provides links to the National Food Safety Initiative; the Office of Women's Health; the Children and Tobacco Web site, which contains tobacco regulation information and also details the effects of tobacco on young people; and MedWatch, a program for the reporting of unsafe medical products by health professionals. Press releases on drug approval are also included on the FDA site.

Health Care Financing Administration (HCFA)
<http://www.hcfa.gov/>

HCFA is responsible for administering the Medicare, Medicaid, and Child Health Insurance programs. This site provides information on qualification criteria, benefits, application procedures, and managed care services for these programs. Information is directed toward consumers and beneficiaries as well as medical care providers and researchers.

Health Resources and Services Administration (HRSA)
<http://www.hrsa.dhhs.gov/>

HRSA "directs national health programs which improve the health of the Nation by assuring quality health care to underserved, vulnerable and special-need populations." This site includes links to the project initiatives and publications of the Office of Minority Health as well as to the HRSA Agenda for Women's Health and Focus on Child Health. The latter site is especially noteworthy for the extensive information it provides on the Healthy Start Program; Healthy Schools, Healthy Communities; Childhood Immunization Initiative; Maternal and Child Health Research Program; Minority Adolescent Health Program; Children's Safety Network; Breastfeeding Initiative; and Traumatic Brain Injury Program.

Indian Health Service (IHS)
<http://www.tucson.ihs.gov/>

The IHS administers health services to American Indians and Alaskan natives belonging to 545 federally recognized tribes. The site provides contact information for area offices and access to publications and reports such as the *Indian Health Manual, State of the Indian Health Service, Trends in Indian Health, Regional Differences in Indian Health*, and *IHS Budget, Spending and Staffing Summary.*

National Institutes of Health (NIH)
<http://www.nih.gov/>

NIH is comprised of twenty-four institutes and centers with responsibility for conducting biomedical research in order "to discover new knowledge that will lead to better health for everyone." NIH Institutes include the National Cancer Institute; the National Eye Institute; the National Heart, Lung, and Blood Institute; the National Institute of Child Health and Human Development; and the National Institute of Arthritis and Musculoskeletal and Skin Diseases. The NIH site includes links to the Health Information Index for assistance in locating the institute within NIH relevant to the specified area of interest as well as links to listings of the most-requested publications by Institute. *The NIH Word on Health*, formerly *HEALTHWise*, is a guide to consumer health information, including topics such as mammograms, untreated ear infections, heart disease, drug-resistant bacteria, antiaging hormones, and Lyme disease.

The Office of Disease Prevention and Health Promotion (ODPHP)
<http://odphp.osophs.dhhs.gov/>

ODPHP's focus is on disease prevention and health promotion, with links to publications such as *Healthy People 2000: Midcourse Review and 1995 Revisions* and *Nutrition and Your Health: Dietary Guidelines for Americans* and to ODPHP coordinated sites, including Healthfinder and the National Health Information Center (NHIC). NHIC's Health Information Resource Database is a subject guide to 1,100 organizations and government agencies that provide health information.

Substance Abuse and Mental Health Services Administration (SAMHSA)
<http://www.samhsa.gov/>

SAMHSA seeks to "improve the quality and availability of prevention, treatment, and rehabilitation services in order to reduce illness, death, disability, and cost to society resulting from substance abuse and mental illnesses." The agency's site links to SAMHSA publications, services, and offices, including the Center for Mental Health Services, the Center for Substance Abuse Prevention, the Center for Substance Abuse Treatment, the Office of Managed Care for mental health and substance abuse services, and substance abuse data from the Office of Applied Studies. The SAMHSA site also promotes the upcoming Surgeon General's Report on Mental Health.

Federal Agencies, Other Than DHHS

Consumer Product Safety Commission (CPSC)
<http://www.cpsc.gov/about/who.html>

This independent agency seeks to "protect the public against unreasonable risks of injuries and deaths associated with consumer products." The scope of the agency's work is outlined and contact information is provided.

Environmental Protection Agency (EPA)
<http://www.epa.gov/>

The EPA seeks to "protect human health and to safeguard the natural environment—air, water, and land—upon which life depends." Information is tailored to specific audiences: researchers and scientists, concerned citizens, students, teachers, children, business, industry, and states. The site provides links to the many and varied EPA programs: acid rain, ozone layer protection, radiation, overexposure to the sun, brownfields, oil spills, endangered species, and the Explorer's Club for children, with information about recycling, protecting the environment for plants and animals, and preventing air and water pollution.

Occupational Safety and Health Administration (OSHA)
<http://www.osha.gov/>

OSHA's mission is to "save lives, prevent injuries and protect the health of America's workers." The site includes an A to Z subject guide to information on topics such as asbestos, indoor air quality, lead, noise and hearing conservation, lead, heat stress, and workplace violence. Also included are links to OSHA publications, including *Job Safety and Health Quarterly*, and to OSHA regulations and compliance-related information.

State Agencies

Council of State Governments (CSG)
<http://www.statesnews.org/>

In existence since 1933, the CSG fosters cooperation and the sharing of ideas and resources between state governments. The site's online publications include *The Health Policy Monitor*, which provides topical articles on health care concerns directed toward state government officials.

National Conference of State Legislatures (NCSL)
<http://www.ncsl.org/>

Designed to assist lawmakers in developing effective policy for state governments, NCSL offers the Health Policy Tracking Service—subscription required—for information on legislative action and tailored reports on specific topics. The site also includes the NCSL Health Issues Web Site, a publicly accessible subject index covering a spectrum of health information.

National Governors' Association (NGA)
<http://www.nga.org/>

NGA is a bipartisan forum for U.S. governors "to establish, influence, and implement policy on national issues." The site includes links to Key State Issues on topics such as maternal and child health, the state children's health insurance program, managed care oversight and quality, and youth development, as well as to NGA Policy Positions and Issue Briefs on domestic issues. NGA Policy Positions includes statements on health care for undocumented immigrants, long-term care, Medicaid, children's health, and managed care and health care reform, among others.

State and Local Government on the Net
<http://www.piperinfo.com/state/states.html>

A user-friendly searchable guide to state and local government, this site provides links to state home pages; statewide offices; legislative, judicial, and executive state branches; state boards and commissions; and city and county home pages for each of the fifty states, in addition to similar information for tribal governments, including American Samoa, Guam, Northern Mariana Islands, Puerto Rico, and the U.S. Virgin Islands.

State Health Departments on the Internet
<http://www.astho.org/html/state_health_agencies_on_the_web.html>

The Association of State and Territorial Health Officials (ASTHO), whose mission is "to formulate and influence sound national public health policy and to assist state health departments in the development and implementation of programs and policies to promote health and prevent disease," maintains this site of links to state health departments.

StateSearch
<http://www.nasire.org/ss/index.html>

StateSearch is a site provided by the National Association of State Information Resource Executives, with links to state government information, including the categories of health, human services, and welfare; state home pages; and state legislatures.

International Agencies

Pan American Health Organization (PAHO)
<http://www.paho.org/>

PAHO is an organization that works to change the health status of its member countries, including eradication of disease, reduction of death from illness, improvement of drinking water supplies and other living conditions, and engagement in health promotion in a variety of areas such as smoking, cancer, cardiovascular disease, and substance abuse. This site identifies the thirty-eight member governments comprising PAHO and provides access to Country Health Profiles for each of the member nations, in addition to information about acquiring PAHO publications.

University of Michigan Documents Center
<http://www.lib.umich.edu/libhome/Documents.center/intl.html>

This site, noted for its comprehensive coverage of government information, also provides extensive links to Web sites on international agencies and information, including those of the American Library Association Government Documents Round Table's International Documents Task Force and the International Organization Web Sites coverage of approximately 4,000 international organizations.

World Health Organization
<http://www.who.int/>

An agency within the United Nations, WHO has 191 member states and has as one of its prime directives "to set global standards for health." This site provides links to information on infectious, tropical, vaccine preventable, and noncommunicable diseases, in addition to topics on health promotion and family and reproductive health. The site also uses Geographic Information System (GIS) applications as part of the HealthMap program to create epidemiological maps for viewing surveillance data on disease control initiatives.

Statistics

CDC Wonder
<http://wonder.cdc.gov/>

CDC WONDER is designed as a "single point of access . . . to public health information for state and local health departments, the Public Health Service, the academic public health community, and the public at large." The site enables querying of numeric data sets in a wide range of subject areas: mortality, cancer incidence, hospital discharges, AIDS, diabetes, fluoridation, fatal accidents, tuberculosis, and others. The site also includes searchable files on chronic disease prevention and cost-benefit/cost-effectiveness studies.

FEDSTATS
<http://www.fedstats.gov/>

The FEDSTATS site is maintained by the Federal Interagency Council on Statistical Policy, with links to statistical information from over seventy federal government agencies. Links to health statistics programs are primarily those of the Department of Health and Human Services. The site includes an A to Z subject guide to statistical information.

National Center for Health Statistics (NCHS)
<http://www.cdc.gov/nchswww/>

NCHS is the premier agency within the federal government with responsibility for collecting, analyzing, and disseminating health statistics. One of the site features is FASTATS, an A to Z subject guide to statistical information that includes data such as annual deaths, age-adjusted death rate, cause of death rank, annual cases, hospital discharges, and average length of hospital stay for particular diseases. Published reports available on the Web site are *Advance Data, National Vital Statistics Reports* (formerly *Monthly Vital Statistics Report), Vital and Health Statistics Series, Vital Statistics of the United States, Health, United States,* and *Life Tables.*

U.S. Census Bureau
<http://www.census.gov/>

Collection of census data every ten years is mandated by the U.S. Constitution. This site provides information about Bureau of the Census reports and publications, including those on health insurance coverage and poverty in the United States. The site also includes an A to Z subject guide to statistical sources and data and the *Report to Congress—The Plan for Census 2000.*

Special Interest Sites

Cool Government Site of the Week
<http://flamestrike.hacks.arizona.edu/~tv/government.html>

This site is an informative, entertaining, randomly updated "interactive civics lesson and guide to the veritable cavalcade of resources available through YOUR government." Current links include information from the Department of Energy on human radiation experiments, the Substance Abuse and Mental Health Services Administration's 1994 National Household Survey on Drug Abuse, and the National Institute for Drug Abuse's guide "Marijuana—Facts for Teens."

GPO Access
<http://www.access.gpo.gov/su_docs/aces/aaces002.html>

A useful site for health policy information, this site provides links to congressional bills, the *Code of Federal Regulations*, the *Congressional Record*, the *United States Code*, the Federal Budget, and the *Federal Register.*

MEDLINEplus
<http://medlineplus.nlm.nih.gov/medlineplus/>

This site, sponsored by the National Library of Medicine, is a selective guide to health information targeted toward consumers. Links are provided to medical dictionaries, health topics on common diseases, physician and hospital directories, and database searching.

National Center for Complementary and Alternative Medicine (NCCAM)
<http://altmed.od.nih.gov/nccam/>

The newly established NCCAM conducts research to determine the effectiveness of alternative medical treatments. The site includes information about program areas and publications with links to the ten specialty research centers funded by NCCAM. The Complementary and Alternative Medicine (CAM) Citation Index allows users to search over 90,000 bibliographic citations, covering the years 1966 to 1997, from the National Library of Medicine's MEDLINE database.

THOMAS
<http://thomas.loc.gov/>

A key resource for legislative—including health policy—information, the THOMAS databases feature searching capabilities by bill number and keyword. Links are provided to the *Congressional Record*; state and local government information; and the legislative, executive, and judicial branches of government.

Resources for Additional Information

Demystifying Documents on the Internet
<http://ublib.buffalo.edu/libraries/units/sel/mkm/michigan/docs.html>

This guide to government Internet resources categorizes searches by the familiar method of known item, subject, agency, statistical, and special techniques with links to relevant resources within each category.

Finding Government Information on the Internet: A Hands on Workshop
<http://www.hazard.uiuc.edu/wmrc/library/govtinfo.htm>

This site features topics such as evaluating Web sites, consumer information, statistics, health sites, and state and local government sources.

Finding Government Information: What's the Difference?
<http://www.libraries.wayne.edu/purdy/govtrain.html>

This site differentiates by type of government information search (title, agency, subject, keyword), with brief listings of links within each category.

How to Effectively Locate Federal Government Information on the Web
<http://gort.ucsd.edu/pcruse/universe/intro.html>

This site explores issues relevant to electronic access to government information and provides links to statistical resources and subject indexes.

REFERENCE NOTES

1. National Library of Medicine to Work with Public Libraries to Help Consumers Find Answers to Medical Questions New Consumer Health Web Site "MEDLINE" Launched. (1998, October 22). *NIH News Advisory* [Online press release]. Available: http://www.nih.gov/news/pr/oct98/nlm-22.htm.

2. Peters, R., and Sikorski, R. "Navigating to Knowledge: Tools for Finding Information on the Internet." *JAMA* 277(February 12, 1997):505-6.

3. Notess, G.R. *Government Information on the Internet.* Lanham, MD: Bernan Press, 1997.

4. Maxymuk, J., ed. *Finding Government Information on the Internet.* New York: Neal-Schuman Publishers, Inc., 1995.

5. Robinson, J.S. *Tapping the Government Grapevine: The User-Friendly Guide to U.S. Government Information Sources.* Third Edition. Phoenix, AZ: The Oryx Press, 1998.

6. Lindberg, D.A.B., and Humphreys, B.L. "Medicine and Health on the Internet: The Good, the Bad, and the Ugly." *JAMA* 280(October 21, 1998):1303-4.

7. Baldwin, G. (1998, May 15). LPS Progress Report. *Administrative Notes: Newsletter of the Federal Depository Library Program* [Online serial], 19(07). Available: http://www.lib.umich.edu/libhome/Documents.center/adnotes/1998/190798/an1907d.txt.

8. Morehead, J. *Introduction to United States Government Information Sources.* Fifth Edition. Englewood, CO: Libraries Unlimited, Inc., 1996.

9. Roper, F.W., and Boorkman, J.A. *Introduction to Reference Sources in the Health Sciences.* Third Edition. Metuchen, NJ: Medical Library Association and Scarecrow Press, Inc., 1994.

10. Maxwell, B. *How to Access the Federal Government on the Internet.* Washington, DC: Congressional Quarterly, Inc., 1997.

11. Maxwell, B. *How to Find Health Information on the Internet.* Washington, DC: Congressional Quarterly, Inc., 1998.

12. Hoben, J.W., ed. *1998 Guide to Health Care Resources on the Internet.* New York: Faulkner and Gray, 1997.

13. Sears, J.L., and Moody, M.K. *Using Government Information Sources Print and Electronic.* Second Edition. Phoenix, AZ: The Oryx Press, 1994.

14. Hersh, W.R. *Information Retrieval: A Health Care Perspective.* New York: Springer, 1996.

SELECTED BIBLIOGRAPHY

Autidore, J., and Stoklosa, K. "Health Statistics Guide to Internet Sites." *College & Research Libraries News* 58(October 1997):627-30.

Breeden, J. II. "HHS Launches HealthFinder." *Government Computer News* 16(1997):8.

Dunn, K. "Web Site: CDC WONDER." *American Journal of Public Health* 87(October 1997):1734-5.

"Finding Your Way." *Patient Care* 31(February 15, 1997):43-4.

Friede, A., and O'Carroll, P.W. "CDC and ATSDR Electronic Information Resources for Health Officers." *Journal of Environmental Health* 59(November 1996):13-22.

Marshall, L. "Health & Medical Industry Research Information on the World Wide Web: A Metasite." *Database* 20(April 1997):57-8.

McCune, J.C. "Ask Uncle Sam: Tapping into Government Web Sites." *Management Review* 86(February 1997):10-11.

Schnell, E.H. "Health and Medicine Web Sites." *The Reference Librarian* (no. 57, 1997):215-22.

Start, N.E. "Health Statistics Sources on the Internet." *Medical Reference Services Quarterly* 16(Spring 1997):1-14.

Thomsen, E. "Health Resources on the World Wide Web." *Collection Building* 17(1998):42-3.

Wilcox, W. ed. *Public Health Sourcebook.* Volume 34. Detroit, MI: Omnigraphics, Inc., 1998.

Chapter 9

Health-Related
Statistical Information on the Net

Dawn M. Littleton
Kathryn Robbins

INTRODUCTION

Health-related statistics are used for a variety of reasons, from justifying public policy and research needs to satisfying personal curiosity. Librarians often say that finding the answers to statistics questions is among the most difficult searches they encounter. This frustration is reflected in the literature: with just one exception, every chapter or article the authors read about finding statistics referred to the inherent challenge and frustration of the search. The good news is that although the accessibility of information on the Net has not eliminated the challenge of finding the particular statistics sought, it has greatly expanded the realm of possible resources to explore.

Many resources already exist that guide seekers to needed statistics. Articles about finding Net-based health statistics are relatively new.[1-4] Even so, descriptions of resources that do not refer to the Internet[5-7] may be useful because many traditional resources have migrated to the easy, inexpensive access of the Internet. This is true especially for the world's largest collector of statistics—the U.S. government.[8] Older descriptions of resources also can enable users to think about the organizations that might collect needed statistics.

When using the Net to find statistical information, two general approaches can be useful:

1. Locate the Net equivalents of print book and journal sources that have proven useful and reliable in the past (e.g., *Statistical Abstract of the United States* at <http://www.census.gov/prod/ 3/98pubs/98statab/cc98stab.htm> and *Morbidity and Mortality Weekly Report* at <http://www.cdc.gov/epo/mmwr/mmwr. html>). They are usually as current or more current than the print versions and can be searched with specific keywords or phrases.

2. Determine who would collect the statistics being sought and who would be likely to share those statistics with the public via the Net. As a general rule, government agencies, at levels from international to local, and nonprofit organizations will be most likely to make their information publicly accessible. For example, if the topic is cancer, the Web sites of the National Cancer Institute and the American Cancer Society are potential places to look. The *Encyclopedia of Associations*[9] is a wonderful resource for finding relevant organizations and includes Web addresses where available.

Four general strategies for finding statistics on the Net are suggested; they are listed here from the most to the least direct:

1. Connect to a recommended Internet address/uniform resource locator (URL). Categories and lists of some of the most well-known addresses for finding health statistics are provided in the next section of this chapter.

2. Utilize a statistics subject list or "metasite" where an individual or group has gathered together many statistics-related Internet sites (e.g., FEDSTATS at <http://www.fedstats.gov/>).

3. Search a bibliographic database (e.g., MEDLINE at <http:// www.ncbi.nlm.nih.gov/PubMed>).

4. If the previous strategies fail, try to find organizations with a search engine or metasearch engine.

Because of the vast array of Internet sites where statistics can be found, it was decided to limit this discussion to those which are freely available on the Net. For discussions of using subscription and pay-as-you-go services to find health statistics (e.g., Dialog and Lexis-Nexis), please see *Finding Statistics Online*.[10] Statistics presented in forms useful for answering ready-reference types of questions were focused upon rather than collections of raw or secondary data (e.g., data files or databanks) that must be analyzed before being used by librarians and consumers. As with all information, whether print or electronic, statistical information on the Net must be critically evaluated for accuracy, authority, and currency.[11,12] Some librarians have raised quality and contextual concerns about health-related statistical information.[1,10]

The following two sections list and briefly describe useful Internet sites for finding health-related statistics. The first category contains statistics based on geographic regions: national, state, metropolitan, and international sources. The second contains sites for special topics: accidents, diseases, health care expenditures, and substance abuse. These sites are described with brief annotations or quotes taken directly from the Internet sites during September 1998.

RECOMMENDED INTERNET ADDRESSES—
GEOGRAPHIC REGIONS

National Statistics

Books

Many books published by the U.S. government have been made available on the Web. Here are some traditional print resources available on the Web.

Greenbook Overview of Entitlement Programs Committee on Ways and Means
<http://aspe.os.dhhs.gov/96gb/intro.htm>

This site "Provides program descriptions and historical data on . . . social and economic topics, including Social Security, employment, earnings, welfare, child support, health insurance, the elderly, families with children, poverty and taxation." The 1994, 1995 and 1996 editions are available.

Health, United States 1998 with Socioeconomic Status and Health Chartbook
Hyattsville, MD, 1998 National Center for Health Statistics
<http://www.cdc.gov/nchswww/products/pubs/pubd/hus/hus.html>

"*Health, United States* presents national trends in health statistics. Major findings are presented in the Highlights. . . . This year socioeconomic status and health was selected as the subject of the chartbook."

Health, United States Series
http://www.cdc.gov/nchswww/products/pubs/pubd/ hus/2010/2010.htm>

From the National Center for Health Statistics, this site contains full texts of the *Health, United States* issues from 1993 to the present. Some issues include a special focus, such as injury (1996-1997) or socioeconomic status (1998).

Healthy People 2000: Midcourse Review and 1995 Revisions
Washington, DC, U.S. Department of Health and Human Services, Public Health Service, 1995
<http://odphp.osophs. dhhs.gov/pubs/hp2000/ midcours.htm>

This site provides a "mid-decade" review of the classic public health book *Healthy People 2000*.

Statistical Abstract of the United States
Washington, DC, Bureau of the Census
<http://www.census.gov/prod/3/98pubs/98statab/cc98stab.htm>

This site not only displays the table of contents of the book but also provides convenient direct links to the entire texts of the 1998, 1997, 1996, and 1995 editions.

Journals

Advance Data From Vital and Health Statistics
<http://www.cdc.gov/nchswww/products/pubs/pubd/ad/ad.htm>

Provided here is early publication of data from the National Center for Health Statistics' health and demographic surveys. Links to issue 254 (August 1994) through the current issue are provided.

MMWR: Morbidity and Mortality Weekly Report
Centers for Disease Control
<http://www.cdc.gov/epo/mmwr/mmwr.html>

This site includes national and state data on notifiable diseases, as well as a review of a selected health problem. Issues include 1982 to present.

Monthly Vital Statistics Report
Hyattsville, MD, U.S. Department of Health, Education and Welfare, Public Health Service, National Center for Health Statistics
<http://www.cdc.gov/nchswww/products/pubs/pubd/mvsrmvsr.htm>

National and state information presenting cumulative and monthly data on births, deaths, marriages, divorces, and infant deaths. The title of this report has changed to *National Vital Statistics Reports (NVSR)* with volume 47, issue 1.

North Carolina Rural Health Research and Policy Analysis Cartographic Archive
<http://www.schsr.unc.edu/research_programs/Rural_Program/maps/maps.html>

This is a useful collection of charts on national health status indicators, health manpower and services, rural areas, and rural hospitals around the United States.

Social Security Agency Office of Research Evaluation and Statistics
<http://www.ssa.gov/statistics/ores_home.html>

Data on old age, survivors, disability insurance, and Supplemental Security Income programs are included here.

Vital and Health Statistics Series (also called "The Rainbow Series")
<http://www.cdc.gov/nchswww/products/pubs/pubd/series/ser.htm>

These ongoing series provide data on many aspects of the national population, including natality and marriage to family growth:

Series 2. Data Evaluation and Methods Research
Series 3. Analytical and Epidemiological Studies
Series 4. Documents and Committee Reports
Series 5. Comparative International Vital and Health Statistics
   Reports
Series 10. Data from the National Health Interview Survey
Series 11. Data from the National Health Examination Survey
   and the National Health and Nutrition Examination Survey
Series 13. Data on Health Resources Utilization; includes
   National Hospital Discharge Survey
Series 14. Data on Health Resources: Manpower and Facilities
Series 15. Data from Special Surveys
Series 20. Data on Mortality
Series 21. Data on Natality, Marriage and Divorce
Series 23. Data from the National Survey of Family Growth
Series 24. Compilations of data on natality, mortality,
   marriage, divorce, and induced terminations of pregnancy

Organizations

Another approach for finding statistics is to think about organizations that will be collecting the statistics being sought and then going to Web home pages. For example, if statistics on accidents are being sought, then those organizations which collect accident data would be likely sources, for example, the National Safety Council and the U.S. government. Health insurance companies probably collect information on accidents, but being private companies, they will be unlikely to share information with the public.

Centers for Disease Control and Prevention (CDC) <http://www. cdc.gov/>

By choosing "Data and Statistics," users can quickly access topics on the "Scientific Data, Surveillance, Health Statistics and Laboratory Information" page. Here disease data can be searched via CDC WONDER (an integration of forty full-text and numeric databases), or more topically in a subject-specific database such as Sexually Transmitted Diseases or the Hazardous Substance Release/Health Effects database. Besides "Scientific Data," there is a section on "Surveillance" that includes access information to the Behavioral Risk Factor Surveillance System, Birth Defects Surveillance, and the HIV/AIDS Surveillance Report.

National Center for Health Statistics (NCHS)
<http://www.cdc. gov/nchswww/>

"NCHS is the primary Federal organization responsible for the collection, analyses and dissemination of health statistics. The intent of this site is to provide users access to the health information that NCHS produces."

U.S. Census Bureau
<http://www.census.gov/main/www/subjects. html>

This site provides many links to general and specific national socioeconomic information, such as age data, characteristics of at-home workers, and population characteristics by zip code.

State Statistics

Many of the national resources already mentioned break down national data into state information. Listed here are additional resources that provide state-level data.

State-Level Data

CDC's "Other health resources on the Internet"
<http://www.cdc.gov/epo/mmwr/medassn.html#states>

These links identify ongoing statewide programs and include helpful contact information.

U.S. Census State Data Centers
<http://www.census.gov/sdc/www/>

This site provides a list of links to the Census State Data Centers that "provide training and technical assistance in accessing and using Census data for research, administration, planning and decision making by the government, the business community, university researchers and other interested data users."

CDC's, Births, STDs, AIDS
<http://www.cdc.gov/nccdphp/dash/ ahson/profiles.htm>

Provided here is information state by state.

Metropolitan Statistics

About 300 metropolitan statistical areas (MSAs) have been defined for the United States. MSAs include core population areas of 50,000 people or more, for example, Los Angeles-Riverside, Orange County, California, and Waterloo-Cedar Falls, Iowa. Data seekers can find details about defined MSAs in *Statistical Abstract of the United States* (described under national resources).

Books

State and Metropolitan Area Data Book 1997-1998
<http://www.census.gov/prod/www/abs/msgen11c.html>

This site includes state and MSA data on births, deaths, physicians, and education.

International Statistics

Books

World Factbook 1997
<http://www.odci.gov/cia/publications/factbook/country-frame.html>

This is the CIA's survey, including brief health statistics, of approximately 200 countries.

Journals

Eurosurveillance Weekly
<http://www.eurosurv.org/main.htm#3>

Updated frequently, this site provides communicable disease surveillance data from European Union public health centers.

Weekly Epidemiological Record (WER)
<http://www.who.ch/wer/>

". . . (WER) serves as an essential instrument for the rapid and accurate dissemination of epidemiological information on cases and outbreaks of diseases under the International Health Regulations, other communicable diseases of public health importance, including the newly emerging or re-emerging infections, non-communicable diseases and other health problems."

Organizations

Demographic and Health Surveys
<http://www.macroint.com/dhs/indicatr/datasearch.asp>

This site is comprised of easily searchable statistics for fertility, childhood mortality, contraception, maternity care, and child health in developing countries.

Epidemiology (Public Health, Biosciences, Medicine), Argus Clearinghouse, by Stephen Shiboski, University of California, San Francisco
<http://www.epibiostat.ucsf.edu/epidem/epidem.html>

Included here is a section on government agencies that provides Web resources by country.

Infonation
<http://www.un.org/Pubs/CyberSchoolBus/infonation/ e_infonation.htm>

This is a searchable database of countries belonging to the United Nations; factors include economy, population, and social indicators.

Pan American Health Organization (PAHO)
<http://www.paho.org/english/country.htm>

"PAHO's country profile database functions as the official regional information source on mortality in the Americas." It includes health profiles of forty-four countries in North and South America.

U.S. Census Bureau's International DataBase
<http://www.census. gov/ftp/pub/ipc/www/idbnew.html>

"The International Data Base (IDB) is a computerized data bank containing statistical tables of demographic and socio-economic data for all countries of the world."

WHOSIS
<http://www.who.ch/whosis/whosis.htm>

This is an extensive resource provided by the World Health Organization that includes many data and full-text resources. Links include access to many topics; "Diseases and Conditions" includes information on child health and development, tropical diseases, noncommunicable diseases, TB, leprosy, and much more.

RECOMMENDED INTERNET ADDRESSES—
SPECIAL TOPICS

Because statistics commonly are sought in several broad areas, such as major diseases or expenditures, useful sources of statistics in these areas are listed in this section. In addition to the specific URLs listed, it is useful to try connecting to a broader "menu" of links or even a search form at the main server address (i.e., the "home page"). To find the home page when a URL is known, successively remove segments of the URL from right to left, back to the next slash and see if that URL proves useful. For example, the Centers for Disease Control and Prevention (CDC) site for AIDS statistics is

http://www.cdc.gov/nchstp/hiv_aids/stats.htm

By removing stats.htm from the URL, the main CDC AIDS Web page will appear:

http://www.cdc.gov/nchstp/hiv_aids/

By removing more of the URL, the CDC home page will appear:

http://www.cdc.gov/

On these higher-level Web pages, searchers can browse provided links or search for appropriate key words.

Accidents

Bureau of Labor Statistics
<http://stats.bls.gov/oshhome.htm>

This is the source for statistics on job-related injuries and illnesses.

Injury Chartbook
<http://www.cdc.gov/nchswww/products/pubs/pubd/hus/2010/2010.htm>

This is the full text of *Health, United States and Injury Chartbook* from the National Center for Health Statistics. It includes injuries by cause, gender, age, geography, and occupation.

National Highway Traffic Safety Administration
<http://www. nhtsa.dot.gov>

This site provides statistics on the number of traffic-related injuries and fatalities, types of vehicles involved in accidents, geographic distribution of accidents, and the searchable Fatality Analysis Reporting System (FARS) database.

National Safety Council
<http://www.nsc.org/lrstop.htm>

This site provides national statistics on the occurrence of accidents (also known as "unintentional injuries"), including some of the tables from the standard reference book *Accident Facts;* it also has some information on the costs associated with accidents.

Diseases

AIDS

CDC—Centers for Disease Control and Prevention
<http://www.cdc.gov/nchstp/hiv_aids/stats.htm>

This site provides links to CDC publications on incidence and trend statistics, most notably the HIV/AIDS Surveillance Report.

Pan American Health Organization (PAHO)
<http://www.paho.org/english/aid/aidepiAe.htm>

"AIDS Surveillance in the Americas Quarterly Reports" contain AIDS incidence and mortality statistics, age, and gender for countries in the Western Hemisphere.

UNAIDS—The Joint United Nations Programme on HIV/AIDS
<http://www.us.unaids.org/highband/fact/index.html>

Fact sheets contain information on the incidence of HIV/AIDS throughout the world, including country-by-country reports of incidence and prevalence.

Cancer

American Cancer Society
<http://www.cancer.org/statmenu.html>

The ACS site provides incidence and trends of the major types of cancer, survival rates, and distribution of cancer by race and ethnic patterns. It includes the full text of *Cancer Facts & Figures.*

Cancer Mondial. International Agency for Research on Cancer (IARC)
<http://www-dep.iarc.fr/>

Included at this site are statistics on cancer incidence, mortality, and survival in many countries throughout the world; coverage is for many years and cancer types.

National Cancer Institute's SEER Program
<http://www-seer.ims.nci.nih.gov>

SEER (Surveillance, Epidemiology and End Results) statistics include cancer incidence, mortality, and survival data from population-based cancer registries in the United States.

Heart Disease

American Heart Association
<http://www.amhrt.org/catalog/Scientific_catpage70.html>

Prevalence and mortality of heart disease and stroke by age, gender, and race are included on this site.

Health Care Costs and Utilization

AHCPR Agency for Health Care Policy and Research
<http://www.ahcpr.gov/data>

This site provides and analyzes data on health care utilization and costs, diagnostic related groups (DRGs), inpatient costs, and principle procedures. It includes ordering information for free publications. Also at the AHCPR site, see the Medical Expenditure Panel Survey (http://www.ahcpr.gov/research/womenmep.htm), which provides data on health status, insurance coverage, health care utilization, costs, and sources of payments.

Bureau of Labor Statistics
<http://stats.bls.gov/oshhome.htm>

This site is the source of health care expenditures by employees and employers, as well as job-related injuries and illnesses.

Health Care Financing Administration (HCFA) Stats and Data
<http://www.hcfa.gov/stats/stats.htm>

HCFA provides data and analysis of recent trends in health care spending, utilization, employment, and prices, both in summary tables and reports (e.g., 1998 Medicare Chart Book) and as public use data files (PUFs).

National Institutes of Health (NIH) Research Funding
<http://www.nih.gov/grants/award/award.htm>

This site includes summaries of funding for health-related research grants and contracts from the National Institutes of Health, including the number and amount of money awarded by city, state, Congressional district, and organization (e.g., university or research institute). See also the summary table of NIH expenditures by disease at <http://www.nih. gov/od/ofm/diseases/index.htm>.

Substance Abuse

National Institute on Drug Abuse (NIDA)
<http://www.nida.nih.gov>

See especially NIDA Infofax (formerly NIDA Capsules) (http://165.112.78.61/Infofax/InfofaxIndex.html).

Substance Abuse and Mental Health Services Administration (SAMHSA)
<http://www.samhsa.gov/oas/oasftp.htm>

This site contains many substantial resources, such as the Substance Abuse and Mental Health Statistics handbook, the National Household Survey on Drug Abuse, Drug Abuse Warning Network (DAWN) reports, and the Treatment Episode Data Set.

METASITES

Metasites are large, well-organized Web sites that provide a browsable list of evaluated resources available on the Web. The major health-related metasites are presented in this book in Chapter 3, "Megasites for Health Care Information." The following is a list of Web guides to statistical resources.

Web Guides to Statistical Resources

BioSites: A Virtual Catalog of Selected Internet Resources in the BioMedical Sciences Statistics
<http://galen.library.ucsf.edu/biosites/ bin/showByTopic. pl?Statistics>

This site provides links to about twenty statistical resources, many already mentioned. It also contains links to statistical information about California.

Health Statistics Page. Falk Library of the Health Sciences— University of Pittsburgh
<http://www.hsls.pitt.edu/intres/guides/statcbw. html>

This is a comprehensive guide that refers users to Web and library resources

Sites with Health Services Research and Public Health Information
<http://weber.u.washington.edu/~hserv/hsic/resource/s-subj. html#sd>

The site consists of links to about twenty-five national or international resources and includes Women's health and an atlas of mortality.

MedWeb Public Health: Vital Statistics
<http://www.gen.emory.edu/MEDWEB/keyword/public_health.html>

Choose either Statistics or Vital Statistics. These different sites contain a small selection of resources ranging from FEDSTATS and local information to dated AIDS mortality to the full text of a health statistics article.

Public Health: HealthWeb. University of Michigan at Ann Arbor, Public Health Library, School of Public Health
<http://www.lib. umich.edu/hw/public.health.html>

This site provides guides to biostatistics, health statistics, and epidemiology.

Statistical Resources on the Web, University of Michigan Documents Center
<http://www.lib.umich.edu/libhome/Documents.center/sthealth.html>

This is an extraordinarily comprehensive directory for statistics on accidents, disability, experimentation, health care, insurance, HMOs, hospitals, life tables, nutrition, substance abuse, transplants, and vital statistics.

Statistics Online: Health
<http://www.berinsteinresearch.com/appfgh.htm#HEALTH>

A comprehensive resource covering many aspects of health care and its finances, this site includes some fee-based resources.

Virtual Library BioSciences—Epidemiology page
<http://chanane.ucsf.edu/epidem/epidem.html>

This site, already mentioned under International Resources, is included here as it has many other types of information; see, especially, Data Sources and Publications.

BIBLIOGRAPHIC DATABASES

Traditional databases can be used to find journal articles containing statistics. Citations in such databases have usually gone through a peer-review process and therefore often lack the bias or commercialism frequently found on Web sites. The drawback is that although citations can be found via the Web, the full-text articles often are not on the Web. Some databases offer access to articles through a document delivery service.

The National Library of Medicine (NLM) provides a number of its journal article databases free over the Internet that previously were available only by subscription. MEDLINE, NLM's premier bibliographic database, indexes monthly thousands of journals in the areas of medicine, nursing, public health and dentistry. It is the online version of three print indexes for health and basic sciences. PubMed (http://www.ncbi.nlm.nih.gov/PubMed/) consists of MEDLINE, some very recent citations that are not yet in MEDLINE, and links to some full-text articles. Internet Grateful Med (http://igm.nlm.nih.gov/) provides access to MEDLINE, HealthSTAR, and many other databases. HealthSTAR indexes articles that discuss effectiveness of programs, products and services, and health care administration and planning. Other databases can be searched by choosing the "Search Other Files" button at the top of the screen. When searching NLM databases for statistical information, expect to employ both subject headings and subheadings.

Both the University of Pittsburgh's Falk Library Health Statistics Web guide[13] and Coates[5] suggest using some of the following subject headings for searching MEDLINE and other NLM databases:

- Birthrate
- Cohort Studies
- Comparative Study
- Cross-Sectional Studies
- Data Collections
- Demography
- Epidemiologic Methods
- Epidemiology Studies
- Factor Analysis, Statistical
- Follow-up Studies
- Incidence
- Longitudinal Studies
- Meta-Analysis

- Morbidity
- Mortality
- Multicenter Studies
- National Center for Health Statistics
- Prevalence
- Probability
- Prospective Studies
- Risk
- Risk Factors
- Statistics
- Vital statistics

In addition to subject headings, it is recommended that subheadings be used. These are generally "attached" to an appropriate disease or nondisease subject heading, but can also be searched independently. Useful subheadings include epidemiology, manpower, mortality, statistics and numerical data, supply and distribution, trends, and utilization. Appropriate subheadings probably are best used in addition to, not in place of, appropriate subject headings. See Chapter 4, "MEDLINE on the Internet," for a more complete discussion of these valuable sources of statistical information.

SEARCH ENGINES

If recommended sites fail to find needed statistics, searchers should consider using Internet search engines (e.g., AltaVista, Hot-Bot, Infoseek) or metasearch engines (e.g., MetaCrawler, Dogpile). Keep in mind that it is often best not to search by the name of the particular statistic (e.g., percent, height, dollars), but by the name of the organization or publication that might report that statistic. Because no one search engine indexes more than 33 percent of the indexable Web, it is a good idea to execute the same search in at least two search engines or a metasearch engine.[14] For more suggestions on the use of search engines, see Chapter 2, "Natural Language and Beyond: Tips for Search Services."

SUMMARY

Searching for a particular statistical fact can be extremely challenging, frustrating, and ultimately rewarding. Some statistics never are found because they never were collected, never were publicly reported, or, in spite of the best skills and intentions, remain undiscovered. If this occurs, and it will on occasion, the search question can be adapted to find the fact that most closely approximates the original information being sought. For example, if the prevalence of diabetes in Ghana seems impossible to find, perhaps finding the incidence in that country will be successful, and, if not, then perhaps available mortality data on diabetes will be suitable.

While the guidelines, suggested approaches, and caveats concerning health statistics described in this chapter should be useful for quite some time, many of the particular URLs listed (as of Summer 1999) undoubtedly will change or cease to exist. However, most of the organizations listed that report statistics will continue to exist, so by finding the new URL of the reporting group and then browsing or searching its new Web site, a data seeker should be on the way to finding needed information.

REFERENCE NOTES

1. Auditore, J., and Stoklosa, K. "Internet Resources: Health Statistics." *C&RL News* 58(October 1997):627-39.

2. Kiley, R. "Health Statistics on the World Wide Web." *Journal of the Royal Society of Medicine* 91(May 1998):264-5.

3. Start, N.E. "Health Statistics Sources on the Internet." *Medical Reference Services Quarterly* 16(Spring 1997):1-14.

4. Wayne-Doppke, J. "Mining the Net for Health Statistics." *Medicine on the Net* 3(May 1997):22-3.

5. Coates, L. "Finding Statistics Online." *Sources* (February 1990):8-10.

6. Weise, F.O., ed. *Health Statistics: An Annotated Bibliographic Guide to Information Resources.* Second Edition. Lanham, MD: Medical Library Association and Scarecrow Press, Inc., 1997.

7. Weise, F., and Johnson, J.M. "Medical and Health Statistics." In F.W. Roper and J.A. Bookman, eds., *Introduction to Reference Sources in the Health Sciences.* Third Edition. Metuchen, NJ: Medical Library Association and Scarecrow Press, Inc., 1994, pp. 203-35.

8. Robinson, J.S. *Tapping the Government Grapevine: The User-Friendly Guide to U.S. Government Information Sources.* Third Edition. Phoenix, AZ: Oryx Press, 1998.

9.   *Encyclopedia of Associations.* Detroit, MI: Gale Research Company. (annual).

10.   Berinstein, P. *Finding Statistics Online: How to Locate the Elusive Numbers You Need.* Medford, NJ: Information Today, Inc., 1998.

11.   Kiley, R. "Quality of Medical Information on the Internet." *Journal of the Royal Society of Medicine* 91(July 1998):369-70.

12.   Silberg, W.M.; Lundberg, G.D.; and Musacchio, R.A. "Accessing, Controlling and Assuring the Quality of Medical Information on the Internet: Caveat Lector—Let the Reader and Viewer Beware." *JAMA* 277(April 16, 1997):1244-5

13.   University of Pittsburgh, Falk Library of the Health Sciences, Health Statistics. <http://www.hsls.pitt.edu/intres/guides/statcbw.html> Accessed: 29 September 1998.

14.   Lawrence S., and Giles, C.L. "Searching the World Wide Web." *Science* 280(April 3, 1998):98-100.

Chapter 10

Electronic Journals on the Internet

Virginia A. Lingle

Medical journals and magazines began as a means for societies and organizations to communicate transactions and other findings among members. Since then, the genre of serial publications has grown to become a significant format in medical libraries for users to access the latest developments in the health sciences. The recent "marriage" of the printed journal with Web technology has again caused a major shift in how users acquire the most up-to-date health information. The concept of electronic access to journal literature involves a wide range of considerations as to scope, format, copyright issues, availability, cost, and much more. This discussion will focus on aspects of Web access to the medical journal literature that would be of interest to the consumer directly or to the health professional assisting a layperson.

SEARCHING THE NET

Numerous Web sites are dedicated to the wide scope of topics related to consumer health—from preventive medicine to alternative therapies to patient advocacy and more. But, how does a person begin a search for health information in electronic journals? Many users start with the search "button" or feature of the Web browser software or Web access service that they are using. The Netscape family of Web-browsing software, for example, leads users to any one of a number of search engines, such as Excite, AltaVista, Go To, Lycos, and others. Search terms or phrases that might be used to find medical information in serial publications could include any combination of the words "consumer" or "patient," "medicine" or "health," "literature" or "journals" or "periodicals" or "magazines" or "serials" or "publications." Usually, these broad search terms result in thousands of "hits" or Web site listings. Browsing through the first few pages of the hit list often produces leads to several useful Web sites that lead to still more links, so that it really is not necessary to scan through thousands of "hits."

The journal resources related to health that are available on the Web are numerous, constantly changing, and extremely varied in complexity and usefulness. The first aspect that a searcher should consider is to clarify exactly what information is being sought— literature written in "everyday" language, professional medical material, or alternative therapies? According to Alan Rees in his fifth edition of *The Consumer Health Information Source Book*, "the number of magazines and newsletters devoted to consumer health is in excess of 150," with only a few achieving circulation in the millions. Most publications focus on specific market segments and have "only a small number of dedicated readers."[1] The breadth of resources continues to broaden when the set of magazines that are written for a nonhealth audience, but include articles on health-related subjects, is considered—magazines such as *Family Circle* or *Women's Day*. As consumers of health services become more sophisticated and knowledgeable, they often are not only looking for literature written for the nonhealth professional but also are seeking the professional, more technical literature. When searching both the lay and professional literature, the challenge of access to the journal literature on the Web takes on a much larger scope, since there are literally thousands of magazine titles related to health and medicine on the market.

Another possible step to searching, then, is to first identify specific names of journals to look for on the Internet rather than using the broad concept of consumer health literature. A user could visit the Web pages of local or regional libraries to view lists of journals subscribed to by a library, if that information is maintained on the Web page, as a way to pinpoint particular magazine titles. The identified titles can then be searched on the Internet to locate specific publisher-created Web pages. Various criteria usually have to be met to access the full text of these journals, but those points will be discussed later. *Prevention Magazine* at <http://healthyideas.com/>, published by Rodale Press, is an example of a publication with an excellent Web site that provides leads to many other useful resources, in addition to selected articles from the journal.

LIBRARY-BASED FILTERS

Rather than searching the entire Internet for individual journal titles, many health sciences libraries have created Web pages with links to electronic resources specifically written for the consumer. Users can often rely on libraries that have already done the work to locate electronic journal Web sites. The Health Sciences Library at the University of Pittsburgh is one library that has an excellent Web page on consumer health at <http://www.hslc.pitt.edu/intres/health/consumer.html> that provides many leads to resources. For example, under the category "Electronic Journals and Newsletters," there is a link to the *Consumer Report's* online service, available to users for $2.95 a month at <http://www.ConsumerReports.org/>. Useful health-related topics at that site range from "Asthma and Air Quality" to "Checking Up On Doctors" to "Mad Cow Disease," even though *Consumer Reports* is not a source that is usually thought to contain health-related information.

Many of the lists of electronic journals available on the Internet have been developed, and are continually maintained by, librarians. The electronic journal list on the Web site of the Countway Medical Library at Harvard (http://www.countway.med.harvard.edu/countway/pubs/pubs.html) is an excellent example of the work being done by libraries. Most titles have restricted access, but some of the titles are accessible by the Internet public. One such title with a free trial period of open access is *Clinical and Diagnostic Laboratory Immunology* (http://cdli.asm.org/), published by the American Society for Microbiology.

Some of the lists initiated by librarians have grown to become major information services with an identity all of their own. The MedWeb service developed by the Emory University Health Sciences Center Library has an extensive Web page with links to electronic publications at <http://www.gen.emory.edu/MEDWEB/

alphakey/electronic_publications.html>. Another service is the New-Jour Web site developed by the University of California at San Diego. Called "the Internet list for new journals and newsletters available on the Internet," it is located at <http://gort.ucsd.edu/newjour/>. This list includes links to journals on all subjects and is not limited to just medicine or consumer health. Another excellent list of links to electronic journals can be found at the Medical Journal Finder site at <http://mjf.de/MJF/MFJ/journalph/ABCframe/frame. html>. Printed lists of Web sites are also available, with one of the best being the *Directory of Electronic Journals and Newsletters,* edited by Diane Kovacs and published by the Association of Research Libraries.[2] An online version is also available. Subscription information for the directory can be viewed at <http://www.arl.org/scomm/edir/97order.html>.

Libraries have also been involved, in many cases, in the development of "metadata" lists of Internet-based resources that include journal lists and other types of links as well. The HealthWeb service at <http:www.healthweb.org/> is an evolving resource developed by the health sciences libraries of the "Big 10+" universities and the Committee on Institutional Cooperation (CIC). Most of the subject specialties profiled include online links or information about journals or magazines related to the subject. The NetWellness site at <http://www.netwellness.org/>, from the libraries at the University of Cincinnati, Case Western Reserve University, and the Ohio State University, has grown into a major information resource for use primarily by citizens of the state of Ohio, but is an excellent example of access to electronic journals for the public that is being developed and maintained by libraries.

As review, a user can begin searching for health-related information in electronic journals by first searching the Internet through a Web browser search engine, such as Excite or Yahoo!, using very general terms with phrases such as "consumer health literature" or "medical electronic journals" to generate a broad list of "hits" to review. Usually, a user only has to browse through the first several pages of the Web sites listed to find leads to other more specific resources. If that technique is not satisfactory, a user can search for the Web sites of medical libraries to find leads to lists of electronic journals for both consumers or health professionals as possible resources. Finally, a user could search for "metadata" lists or filters that often include leads to electronic journals. Libraries have been in the forefront in the development of such lists, as have physicians and other health professionals and the U.S. government, as explained in the following sections.

PHYSICIAN-DEVELOPED FILTERS

Other lists of electronic journals have been developed by physicians and health professionals to organize access to the medical literature. One example is the WebMedLit Web site at <http://www.webmedlit.com/>. Promoted as a means to provide "efficient access to the best medical journals on the Web," the service is sponsored by Silver Platter Information, Incorporated, and Physicians' Home Page. WebMedLit tracks twenty-two core medical journals by listing the latest table of contents for each title. Clicking on the article title will lead the user to the publisher's Web site for the journal, which may or may not allow access to the full text depending on the user's registration status. Some publishers will load the full text of selected articles at no charge for a limited period of time. Medical Matrix at <http://www.medmatrix.org> is another Web site that tracks the medical literature. A third example of a physician-developed Internet site is YourHealth.com at <http://www.yourhealth.com/>, which provides access to the "MDX Health Digest" service. Users can search a database of references to articles from a mix of professional and consumer literature ranging from the *Annals of Internal Medicine* to *McCall's* to *The Washington Post Health* publication. Summaries or abstracts of the content are provided for every reference.

GOVERNMENT FILTERS
TO ELECTRONIC JOURNALS

The U.S. government is probably the largest producer of consumer health information in the world. Several Web-based lists of electronic journals are maintained by health-related departments. The Department of Health and Human Services has produced healthfinder at <http://www.healthfinder.org/>, which includes an

"Online Journals" page listing over sixty-five professional and consumer health journals. One title included on this list that has full text available for free is *Complementary and Alternative Medicine* at http://altmed.od.nih.gov/nccam/cam/.

The major government resource for information about medical journals, however, is the MEDLINE database, produced by the National Library of Medicine at the National Institutes of Health in Bethesda, Maryland (see Chapter 4, "MEDLINE on the Internet," for detailed information). Since the 1970s, MEDLINE has usually been the first tool that medical librarians use to search the medical literature, and now MEDLINE is available to the public at no charge through the PubMed Web site <http://www.nih.nlm.gov/PubMed/>. Many other Web sites also package access to the MEDLINE database. One example is HealthWorld Online at <http://www.healthy.net/>.

In MEDLINE, users can search citations to the professional medical journal literature. References include authors, article title, journal name, volume, pages, and date of publication, in addition to abstracts or paragraphs summarizing the article content for over 50 percent of the references. MEDLINE through PubMed also includes links to the publisher Web sites to access the full text of articles for many of the journals.

A version of the Web site tailored for consumers is called MEDLINE*plus* and includes links to dictionaries, clearinghouses, directories, and online publications as well as the full MEDLINE database. The online publications include government documents, online newsletters and magazines, electronic books, and health news resources. The *JAMA Patient Page* by the American Medical Association (AMA), which is included in the health news listing on MEDLINE Plus, leads readers to selected full-text articles from the magazine.

ASSOCIATION-DEVELOPED LISTS

Web pages developed or sponsored by professional health-related organizations, societies, or associations are often a direct link to their publications. Some sites offer full-text access to their journals as part of membership benefits, or the organization may actually load the full text of selected articles from their journals and make them available to the Internet public for a limited time. One of the most significant examples of this type of service is the American Medical Association (AMA) Web site at <http://www.ama-assn.org/>. The AMA provides access to their journal publications at various levels, including table of contents with abstracts, selected full-text articles available at no charge, complete full-text access of some of their publications (*MSJama* for medical students), document delivery options through the Carl UnCover service, and promotion of subscriptions to both the print and online full text.

The *Journal of Orthomolecular Medicine* at <http://www.healthynet/library/journals/>, the official journal of the International Society for Orthomolecular Medicine, provides free full-text access for the most current issue and makes reprints of older articles available at $2.50 per article using a secure online credit card transaction system. Another example is the American Psychological Association (APA), which publishes a number of professional journals and provides the full text of its publication *APA Monitor Online* (http://www.apa.org/monitor/), in addition to a wealth of information for the public related to psychology, at its Web site. Many of the association Web sites include useful features, such as medical meeting information or links to other related Web resources.

OTHER PRODUCERS OF ELECTRONIC JOURNAL LISTS

In addition to the groups already mentioned, it seems that every type of information-providing entity is represented on the Internet with its own Web page. Producers of electronic journals, magazines, or newsletters can include individuals, companies selling products, professional organizations/societies/associations, hospitals, medical centers, research centers, drug companies, advocacy groups, individual health care providers or medical practice sites, publishing companies, foundations, and even health sciences libraries. Web pages developed by individuals may be useful, but often the content is the "this is my story and what works for me" type of information and is not authoritative health information. One exception is a very useful guide developed by Judy Bakstran, a consumer searching for information about her husband's cancer. Her Web site, titled "The Guide to Medical Information and Support on the Internet" at <http://www.geocities.com/HotSprings/1505/guide.html>, includes links to mainstream organizations and publications.

Company Web pages are usually developed to sell products and may contain a company newsletter or links to other publications. However, unique medical information companies have emerged that provide free use of resources for the Internet public. One source of funding for these sites seems to be advertising that flashes on the screen as the browser is accessing the service. An example of one such company is Mediconsult at <http://www.mediconsult.com>, which includes links to journal article citations. This service also provides expanded abstracts, that is, longer summaries than are usually found, plus a series of questions and answers supplied by the author to further explain the article content. Online links to organizations relevant to the content are frequently included.

Another excellent service is Medscape at <http://www.medscape.com>. The service is free but requires registration. Once a user has a password, numerous resources can be accessed. The "Journals" section of the site allows "free access to Medscape's own collection of over 25,000 full-text articles. In addition, complete access to all medical journals in Dow Jones Interactive Publications Library on a pay-per-view basis" is available. Full-text articles can be downloaded from over thirty-nine medical journals, including *Diabetes Care*, published by the American Diabetes Association, Incorporated; the *Journal of the American Board of Family Practice; Nutrition and Cancer*, published by Lawrence Erlbaum Associates, Incorporated; and the *Southern Medical Journal*.

As part of increased competition for patients, many medical centers, hospitals, and research centers are also promoting services for the consumer, including access to their own journal literature. The Health Oasis service, produced by the Mayo Clinic (http://www.mayohealth.org/mayo/common/html/), provides access to "articles" on common health topics such as cancer, nutrition, and women's health, for example.

Publishing companies, of course, are the largest providers of electronic journal information on the Internet because, in most cases, they own the journal content. Web-based access to online journals is constantly changing as the companies continue to experiment with cost-recovery options and user demand. Initially, many publisher-based systems made full text available to only library consortiums that also had a strong base of print subscriptions to the same journals, but as electronic access to journals continues to evolve and consumer demand continues to grow, publishers are developing access options for individual or personal subscriptions as well. The larger publisher-based services include the IDEAL system from Academic Press at <http://www.apnet.com>; Elsevier's Science Direct service at <http://scienceserver.orionsci.com>; Highwire Press at <http://highwire.stanford.edu>; the Institute of Physics Electronic Journals service at <http://www.iop.org>; Project Muse of the Johns Hopkins University Press at <http://muse.jhu.edu>; and the LINK service by Springer-Verlag at <http://link.springer-ny.com>.

CHALLENGES OF ACCESS
TO ELECTRONIC JOURNALS FOR CONSUMERS

There are a number of challenges to accessing the electronic journal literature to find quality health-related information. Some of the aspects are inherent in the nature of the Internet itself, whereas others are more specific. In general, the obstacles to access revolve around the issues of who provides the information, who may use the various services, what content is included, and what is the quality of the information being provided. Consumers and health science library professionals assisting consumers need to consider the following factors when searching the Web for reliable health information in a journal format.

User Authorization or Registration

Authorization to access electronic journals can take many forms. Some Web sites require users to register for a password and user ID that will be assigned by the service and then sent to the user either by electronic mail or regular mail. With some sites, a user can assign his or her own user ID and password. It's always a challenge to remember personal login ID numbers, so an individual should try to use the same password with every registration, if possible. There are journals that have full text available with "no strings attached"—no special login or authorization required to establish access—but these are relatively few in number. Hirewire Press is one of the first companies to have provided access to medical journals for free as part of a trial project with no special registrations needed. Some sites load the full text of the most current issue and/or selected articles of a journal, but do not allow access to the full text of back issues unless a subscription fee is paid.

In the mid-1990s, the trend with several publishers was to load the full text of selected journals as part of a pilot project to test their own proprietary Web access systems. The Springer LINK system and the IDEAL system by Academic Press are two examples of such projects. The Karger and Wiley companies have also developed their own Web sites to access the journals that they publish. Initially, electronic access was free and available to the entire Internet public, but the next phase in development was to add some requirement to access—either password registration or proof of a subscription to the print version of the title, such as a subscription confirmation number, in order to access the electronic journal. Most recently, the trend is for publishers to charge a slight percentage above the print subscription price to add Web access capabilities. Some publishers even require that in order to maintain a print subscription, a combined print-online price must be paid, and there is no option to purchase the print format alone.

Free access to the full text of some electronic journals is still available on the Web, but often, these resources are newsletters or publications that are subsidized by advertising or organizational sponsorship. More companies are requiring a payment or some type of commitment, such as an organization membership, that is defined in a contract or "statement of agreement" outlined on the Web site.

User Agreements

Access to the full-text level of journals often involves a contract or some terms of an agreement. When submitting identification information online to subscribe or register for a title, some suppliers display the conditions for access with no option to negotiate or change them. A user must either click on the agree "button" or the registration is not completed and access is denied. A statement of agreement for access should be reviewed very carefully. Some of the conditions for which journal publishers require compliance include use of the service within the bounds of the copyright law; authorized functions such as searching, displaying, copying, and downloading articles; and specified payment and renewal terms. The Association of Research Libraries has published a pamphlet that provides useful guidelines to individuals considering access to electronic journals. Titled "Licensing Electronic Resources: Strategic and Practical Considerations for Signing Electronic Information Delivery Agreements,"[3] it is available full text on the Web at <http://www.arl.org/scomm/licensing/licbooklet.html>. Libraries that register for access to electronic journals wrestle with each of the points mentioned here as well as others, such as interlibrary loan use, simultaneous user access, and connections from multiple geographic locations.

Quality or Level of Content

Much of the assessment of an electronic journal is very similar to the criteria that would be used to evaluate the quality of a printed journal. A user looking for health-related information on the Internet should be asking many questions. Always judge the resource according to the validity or reputation of the producer of the publication. Does the information seem to be correct and reliable? Is the producer of the information established and well known, such as the American Medical Association or the Mayo Clinic? Another point that should be considered is whether the cost of accessing the information is worth the product. Could the same information be obtained elsewhere for free or at a lower cost? When was the information produced? Is there a publication date or some indication that the information is up to date? When was the last date that the Web site was updated? If the last update was several years ago, the validity of the information may be in question. Is the information on a specific topic easy to find on the Web site? Does the magazine have its own search feature to easily locate resources, or must a user browse through a complicated list of subjects or numerous pages of content? Does the electronic journal have a link to the National Library of Medicine's PubMed MEDLINE Web site so that individual articles can be located by first searching that database? What level of information is actually provided in the electronic journal? Does it include text and pictures or charts? Is the content written in easy-to-understand terms, or is the information highly technical?

Electronic journals on the Web can be as varied in content as their print counterparts, if not more so. Some sites are mostly promotional advertisements for printed versions of a title, whereas others are only available full text online with no print counterpart on the market. Some electronic journals include interactive features that are in addition to, or part of, journal articles, such as an online "ask the doctor" service or an online "body mass index" calculator or calorie counter, for example. A document delivery service may be provided by a journal Web site, as is the case with the magazine *Aids Weekly Plus* (http://www.newsfile.com/xla.htm). Readers can click on titles of articles in the table of contents to view a brief summary paragraph, and they then have the option to click on a button to select the article for purchase directly from the publisher. Another document delivery service is the Carl UnCover Web site at <http://uncweb. carl.org>, which is a very user-friendly and reasonably priced resource from which to order reprints or copies of articles from the health-related literature, as well as journals and magazines in many subject areas.

The coverage or content of electronic journals can also vary by the date of material that is included. Medical publishers began to experiment with Web site content in the early 1990s. The Ovid company loaded content for some journals beginning with 1993 issues. Many electronic versions of publications have only become available in the mid-1990s, with producers giving no indication of loading retrospective years online. What remains to be seen for the user is whether companies or journal providers will retain content that has been made accessible online or whether early years will be deleted to "make room" for the more recent years.

SHIFTING TRENDS

The provision of electronic journals on the Internet has made a major impact on the publishing industry, and providers will continue to see a transition in how people access the information they need—health related or otherwise. Increasingly, Web-based full-text information is available on the Internet, not in the familiar format of a journal or magazine or even a newsletter, but as separate narratives or collections of "articles" by subject. More frequently, there is no volume number or issue number or even date attached to the information. A recent issue of *Nature* magazine contained a very stimulating and thought-provoking article about journals on the Web titled "The Writing Is on the Web for Science Journals in Print."[4] The same outlook may be true for all types of magazines, not only the science literature. Consumer health information on the Internet, particularly, is evolving from familiar print formats to more interactive packaging. A Web site may include question-and-answer feedback pages that tailor the information received by the user according to a personal profile or other data that are supplied by the consumer. The information retrieved may be in the form of a "patient handout sheet" or full-text explanation written by health professionals without the framework of being part of a magazine. Web sites produced by traditional magazine publishers are increasingly including other services or links along with the electronic journal that add to the transition away from the traditional print format. The key word is "transition." Currently, information is becoming increasingly accessible in all formats, as journal producers of all kinds continue to load publications on the Internet, for free or otherwise; as librarians and other professionals attempt to organize what is available with more user-friendly interfaces; and as the consumer becomes more sophisticated and demanding of valid medical information on the Internet.

REFERENCE NOTES

1. Rees, A.M. *The Consumer Health Information Source Book*, Fifth Edition. New York: Orxy Press, 1998, p. 46.

2. Kovacs, D. *Directory of Electronic Journals and Newsletters.* Washington, DC: Association of Research Libraries, 1998.

3. Brennan, P.; Hersey, K.; and Harper, G. *Licensing Electronic Resources: Strategic and Practical Considerations for Signing Electronic Information Delivery Agreements.* Washington, DC: Association of Research Libraries, January 1997, 23 pp.

4. Butler, D. "The Writing Is on the Web for Science Journals in Print." *Nature* 397(January 21, 1999):195-200.

Chapter 11

Searching International Medical Resources on the World Wide Web

Jeri Ann Risin

THE BARRIERS TO INTERNATIONAL RESEARCH

The gathering of information from international resources has always proven a unique challenge, regardless of the country out of which the research efforts were based. The obstacles to effective information gathering are always the same: Languages may be spoken, as well as written, in a form we do not understand. Cultural differences may cause misunderstandings and misinterpretations.

When searching for health and medical information on an international level, additional problems may arise. Because geographical, lifestyle, and environmental factors all contribute to our general health status, we find that some medical issues vary in importance from place to place. Therefore, different areas of the world may not provide satisfactory medical information about a certain epidemic or condition simply because it is not common enough to promote significant research attention there. Not only this, but a number of countries in the world today are still developing their economies, technologies, networks, and communications abilities. These countries may have valuable health and medical information to share, but are not yet able to do so.

USING THE WORLD WIDE WEB TO BREAK DOWN THE BARRIERS

As the world's largest online network, the Internet can supply timely information to a great number of individuals at dispersed geographical locations. As we know, the use of the World Wide Web has promoted communications and exchanges of information in all fields.

The World Wide Web has certainly facilitated our ability to locate health and medical information on an international level. Organizations supporting the dissemination of international medical data, which have been in existence long before the Web, have been able to establish their accessibility as never before. Not only this, but new organizations promoting the sharing and distributing of international health and medical information have formed because of the presence of the World Wide Web. Cultural and language barriers have become secondary in many of these cases because the mission of these organizations is the same: to promote global health and medical information sharing and distribution on a collaborative level worldwide.

The Internet Web sites you will learn about in this chapter are a reflection of both the long-existing organizations that now have a Web presence and those which have come into existence because of the World Wide Web. All offer health and medical data in the English language. Also, the majority of the information you will find on them is immediately accessible and free. The sites cover either global or regional medical information rather than focusing on medical data from one specific country. Because it is recognized that certain areas of the world are restricted by poor communications and economic conditions, and hence are not usually known to offer a lot of significant medical data, sites that emphasize information from these countries have been included. Various health and medical issues are the focus. The purpose here is to provide access to various medical topics of interest on an international level, while overcoming the barriers typical to international research.

INTERNATIONAL MEDICAL INFORMATION RESEARCH SITES ON THE WORLD WIDE WEB

Healthnet

SatelLife uses a combination of technologies, such as microsatellites, telephone lines, and surface radio, to link health care workers together in a computer-based electronic network. Through its computer network, Healthnet, SatelLife provides information services to health professionals, principally in developing countries. Healthnet is operational in over thirty countries in Africa, Asia, and Latin America. Its estimated user base of 4,000 has access to e-mail, current health information, electronic discussion groups, and other services. SatelLife focuses on the improvement of communications and exchanges of information in the fields of public health, medicine, and the environment, placing a special emphasis on areas of the world where access is limited by poor communications, economic conditions, or disasters.

SatelLife Healthnet creates access to timely, high-quality health information worldwide. It does this in two ways. First, it features a number of informative links; second, it provides a searchable database that contains profiles of health professionals around the world with whom you may network via e-mail.

Many of Healthnet's informative links are either to SatelLife's own resources or to those of sponsors who have collaborated with Healthnet. One SatelLife resource is its "Health Statistics at a Glance." For a number of countries, you may locate a quick snapshot of some of their health statistics, such as population, people per physician, and life expectancy.

ProCOR: Healthnet has collaborated with several sponsors to create other valuable sources of information at its site. In a collaborative effort between the Lown Cardiovascular Center and SatelLife, an international electronic conference of emerging cardiovascular diseases called ProCOR is present. ProCOR offers a platform for the exchange of information and the engagement of dialog related to cardiovascular health issues in the developing world. Its features include the following:

- A moderated discussion group
- A section of landmark articles in full text related to the diagnosis, therapy, or prevention of cardiovascular disease
- A forum for scientists and health care workers to post and discuss their research activities
- Monthly commentary by an invited editorial presenting the views of leading experts and members of ProCOR's advisory

committee on topics of special importance to cardiovascular
health in developing countries
- Literature abstracts of important recent articles
- Most important papers of the year published in full text

The SatelLife Healthnet Database of Health Professionals contains profiles of HealthNet users and other health professionals.
Registration is free, and once you have done so, you may search the
database to find a colleague who shares the same professional interests as yourself. You may then contact that person by e-mail and
perhaps exchange ideas, data, and expertise with persons halfway
around the world. You may choose to make your profile searchable
by others so that colleagues may also locate and contact you.

Aside from the database of health professionals, you may also
communicate with colleagues through discussion groups. A number
of separate discussion groups cover many different topics, including injury surveillance control and intervention, pediatric respiratory medicine, the Program for Monitoring Emerging Diseases, epidemiology, and drugs.

SatelLife Healthnet also uses e-mail to distribute a number of
electronic publications, such as the AIDS Daily Summary and the
WHO Library Digest for Africa. For each publication, an "info file"
exists that will contain information describing the publication and
how to subscribe to it. You may use e-mail to retrieve the "info file"
for any of the publications available.

There is a "Clips & Quotes" section on this site, also. This area
contains special articles and reports featuring new health information resources that can be found on the Internet.

When you visit the site, it may be a good idea to browse through
the SatelLife Healthnet Information Services Guide. You may locate its link on the SatelLife home page. The guide will explain the
full range of services available from SatelLife and how you may
access them and use them to your benefit.

Also on the home page, you will notice a link to a search engine
in the lower right corner. SatelLife uses WebGlimpse to search its
site. Glimpse is an indexing and querying system that is capable of
searching large indexes quickly. You may enter a search string for a
medical topic of interest along with some other criteria. Your query

will return results in both full text and bibliographic citations. Results from a search of the SatelLife site will include articles, conference proceedings, papers, and so forth.

Demographic and Health Surveys
<www.macroint.com/dhs>

The Demographic and Health Surveys program is funded primarily by the U.S. Agency for International Development. It features one of the world's largest primary information sources pertaining to men, women, and their families residing in Africa, Asia, Latin America, and the Caribbean. DHS collaborates with institutions in developing countries to conduct national surveys on fertility, family planning, child health, maternal health, and household living conditions.

DHS allows you to build customized data tables about mortality rates, fertility, child health, and maternity for individual countries or regions of the world. Data tables include the relevant statistics and the size of the sample surveyed.

Following the publication of results from a DHS survey or research study, a news release is written. The news release helps the Demographic and Health Surveys program communicate the research results in ways that will strengthen understanding and use of the data. Their purpose is to back up the information with narrative text. News releases are organized by country.

DHS offers an online catalog of its publications, most of which are sent to regional depositories, organizations, and libraries involved in the subject areas of population, family planning, and maternal and child health. The publications are arranged by type: final reports, summary reports, comparative studies, and so on, each with its own hypertext link. The links usually lead to a site that provides ordering information or perhaps a bibliographic listing of titles available within that publication type. However, the DHS Newsletter link will take you to a sampling of full-text newsletter articles.

If you are interested in reviewing the other projects of interest at DHS, look under the "News" section on the home page. This section will tell you about current surveys in progress and provide survey excerpts.

The Demographic and Health Surveys home page features hypertext links that will take you to all the major areas, such as the News area, the Statistics area, and the Publications and Manuals area. This site is also relatively easy to navigate.

Outbreak
<www.outbreak.org>

Outbreak is an online information service that focuses on emerging diseases around the globe. It acts as a collaborative database that tracks information about outbreak events worldwide. Outbreak also provides a general overview of emerging diseases and issues related to the emergence of multiple-drug-resistant disease strains.

Many resources are available at the Outbreak site. The major sections include an overview of emerging diseases, in-depth information about specific emerging diseases, and information about currently active and historical outbreaks.

The emerging diseases section provides detailed coverage of such diseases as ebola, malaria, monkeypox, and yellow fever. When a disease is selected, a table of contents page for information about the disease appears, along with a list of links to the latest news about it. Sections in the table of contents cover Frequently Asked Questions; Scientific developments; People and Interviews; History; the Media; and Resources. All of the information here is in full-text format and is taken from a wide variety of resources around the globe. Information for each disease is provided using a common format. Some of the information elements in the format include an FAQ (frequently asked questions) document; pictures and movies of the involved bacteria, viruses, transmission vectors, and symptoms; basic prevention recommendations; basic treatment recommendations; and information about vaccines.

The overview section of emerging diseases, titled "General Information," offers articles and essays about emerging diseases, reports on current outbreaks, a reading list of books, and a resource center that lists links to related sources from WHO, *Morbidity and Mortality Weekly Report*, and so on.

At this writing, the Outbreak Channel is a brand-new feature on this site. This service requires the new version 4 browser of Microsoft Internet Explorer. The Outbreak Channel features push technology, allowing you to receive updated Outbreak content and news directly on your desktop on a continuous and regular basis.

The diseases at this site have been selected based on the degree to which they capture the attention of the general public, make an impact on daily human life, and cause unique emergence issues, such as multiple drug resistance.

There are hundreds of pages of information at this site. You may want to look at the Outbreak FAQ document in the welcome section on the Outbreak home page. This document will tell you more about Outbreak in general, including the accuracy of their resources. You may also check the First Time Visitors section. The guide will explain how Outbreak is organized, as well as give you the key to certain symbols you will see connected to the information found at this site. There is certainly a lot of data here, but the home page organizes the links to it in a logically structured order. Also, at the bottom of most pages, you will notice a menu of links that you can use to transfer to different sections of Outbreak.

World Health Organization
<www.who.org>

The objective of the World Health Organization (WHO) is to assist all peoples in the attainment of the highest possible level of health. To support this mission, WHO covers a wide range of functions and conducts extensive programs in the treatment and prevention of disease. WHO covers regions from all over the globe: Africa, Americas/ Pan America, Eastern Mediterranean, Europe, Southeast Asia, and the Western Pacific.

At its Web site, WHO has grouped its information into several categories, including What's New, Governance, Health Topics, and Information Sources.

If you enter the Health Topics section, you will be able to select from a list. By selecting a disease, you will most likely be transferred to a page that features a WHO program for that disease, if there is one. Also, you will be given links to news and other information resources pertaining to that disease. For example, if you select POLIO as your health topic, you will be linked to the Global Programme for Vaccines and Immunizations page. A sidebar will show you links to News, Polio Eradication, Diseases & Vaccinations, and Documents. The information provided via the links includes updates on progress made on the disease around the globe, statistics on the disease, and a world prognosis for the disease.

The Press Material area will link you to WHO press releases and fact sheets. The fact sheets, which are accessible here in full text, contain factual information for all regions of the world on various health topics, such as blindness, child mortality, food-borne diseases, health promotion, Parkinson's disease, and sanitation.

The Information Sources section will provide access to WHO documentation, such as background information on WHO, WHO publications, WHO policies documents, and health-related Web servers. This section will also give you access to such resources as World Health Reports, WHO collaborating centers' Web pages, and contact information to the WHO headquarters directory.

The Information Sources section also features access to WHO-SIS (WHO Statistical Information System). WHOSIS provides statistical and epidemiological data and information presently available from WHO and elsewhere in electronic or other forms. For example, WHO has a database called Health for All that is downloadable directly from its Web site. Health for All is full of worldwide statistical indicators for all kinds of health information, all of which is searchable. Searches can be performed by selecting countries (or groups of countries), indicators, and years. Indicators include numbers of doctors, numbers of beds, salaries of health personnel, GNP expenditures, incidences of selected diseases, death rates of selected diseases, maternity statistics, vitality statistics, population, and so forth. Results may be viewed as a total global number or as a statistic for a specific country. The results can be displayed on one of two different table formats or can be charted on two different kinds of graphs. In addition, they can be downloaded onto a spreadsheet program. The cost of the database is currently free, if you elect to download it from the Web.

Another way of finding and using data on WHOSIS is to search WHO information by disease topic. From a list of links, you may select either a disease or a general topic, such as food safety. You will probably then find yourself linked to a page that features a program for the disease or topic you chose and be able to use sidebar links to access further data.

Besides downloadable databases and links to statistics and epidemiology, WHOSIS offers selected statistical tools and applications useful for working with such data. You may link to the International Classification of Diseases or download the Johns Hopkins Delta Omega, which is public domain software for public health.

WHO offers a site map that you may link to from its home page to help you find your way. The site map will group WHO topics together by categories of information source types or by subjects of interest. You may also use the WHO search engine, found at the bottom of the home page, to locate information. This site is full of hypertext links that are cross-referenced in many places. The links are logically connected and arranged, making it easy to pinpoint an area of interest. Although the site is comprehensive, you can steer your way through it smoothly because of the link structure. However, because WHO is a vast organization, there are many other Web sites of interest connected to it. It may be a good idea to prioritize ahead of time what part of WHO you would like to concentrate on, whether it be a particular WHO-related organization, country, disease, or topic.

Center for International Health Information
<www.cihi.com>

The purpose of CIHI (Center for International Health Information) is to provide timely, reliable, and accurate information on the population, health, and nutrition of developing countries, assisted by the U.S. Agency for International Development.

Readily available at CIHI's Web site are statistical indicators for population, health, and nutrition by region. Currently, the regional summaries are offering four different focus areas: infant mortality rates, under-five mortality rates, total fertility rates, and contraceptive prevalence rates.

CIHI also offers its Country Health Profile Series, which is accessible as full-text statistical reports with multiple indicators. Reports are available as text or PDF (portable document format) files. These reports cover most of the individual countries located in Africa/Sub-Sahara, Asia/Near East, Latin America, and the Caribbean. Soon to come will be the Eastern European region and the newly independent states.

The CIHI publications area provides full-text access to staff analysis and reports. As of this writing, there were only a few reports available in this section.

CIHI also provides links to other health resources on the Web, including the United Nations, WHO, World Bank, Japanese International Cooperation Agency, British Overseas Development Administration, various foreign Ministries of Health, and international Internet guides, such as the Global Health Network.

The CIHI site is fairly easy to navigate. Each section of information is listed as a link on a sidebar at the home page. Once you have transferred to the area of interest, you will be provided with a description of the information there, and you will see links to take you to your topic.

PharmWeb
<www.pharmweb.net>

PharmWeb contains comprehensive international pharmaceutical information provided by professional organizations. It is a one-stop source of pharmaceutical resources, including conferences, pharmaceutical job openings, discussion forums, patient information, professional contacts, government and regulatory data, educational opportunities, and worldwide organizations.

The PharmWeb home page lists the contents of the site by major category groupings. Categories include PharmWeb Chat, Patient Information, Worldwide Pharmacy Colleges/Departments/Schools, and Societies. For a considerably more detailed breakdown of the site's contents, refer to the site index, which lists all available topics in alphabetical order. Access to the sponsors' Web pages is also featured on the home page.

Each of the major category groupings will lead to live, full-text, ready-to-use documents. For example, the Patient Information link leads the user to information on how to use medicines and provides access to a guide on how to treat common ailments with pharmaceuticals. The Conferences and Meetings link leads to Web pages of various pharmaceutical conferences. If it is important to remain updated on pharmaceutical information in various parts of the world, PharmWeb features a mailing list via the PharmWeb World Drug Alert link. Users may select to receive country-specific information via e-mail about topics such as product recalls or drug interactions. The choice of country is up to the user to select, as is the topic.

PharmWeb also features a directory to manufacturers, clinical trials, diagnostics, journals, and so on. The directory is located via the PharmWeb Yellow Pages link and provides access to information via a hypertext list of major headings and a search engine.

The search engine on PharmWeb is called PharmSearch and allows searches by keywords, separated by a space. Results produce links to press releases, programs, and Web pages. English is not the only language featured on this site, so some links are to foreign-language Web pages.

There are three ways to explore this site. The first is by browsing through the home page categories, which feature all the major areas of the site. The second way is by going to the comprehensive site index and browsing the detailed topic listings in alphabetical order. Last, the search engine is a good feature to use for direct keyword searches.

OTHER SITES OF INTEREST

The following is a brief summary of some other places to visit on the World Wide Web that offer access to international medical information resources.

Medical Schools Around the World

Medical Schools Worldwide
<www.geocities.com/Athens/Acropolis/7895/index.html>

This is a clickable graphic map of the world. If you click on a continent, a list of links to medical school Web sites in that region appears.

Medical Schools
<www.med.ualberta.ca/links/medlinks/school.html>

This site contains a list of regions of the world; you will be linked to a list of medical school Web sites that are within each region.

Medical Bank Institute—World Medical Schools
<www.medbank.or.jp/home/desc460.html>

This site contains an alphabetical list of links to medical schools around the world. About 70 percent of the schools are in the United States.

Drugs and Pharmaceutical Information

Worldwide Drugs
<community.net/~neils/new.html>

This is a starter page to access international Internet sites that provide drug and pharmaceutical information.

DrugText
<www.drugtext.nf>

This site contains full-text information on substance abuse and drug usage in countries around the world. It includes access to articles, press releases, organizations, and country-specific drug policies.

International Pharmaceutical Federation
<www.pharmweb.net/pwmirror/pw9/fip/pharmweb92.html>

This site covers resources about pharmaceutical science. It includes newsletters, a list of pharmacy schools around the world, organizations, conferences, and so forth.

Medical Literature in Full Text

BOPCAS—British Official Publications Current Awareness Service
<www.soton.ac.uk/~bopcas/>

Records of the new United Kingdom official publications from July 1995 to present can be accessed here. Health and medical topics are included.

Helen L. Deroy Medical Library—Full Text Electronic Journals
<www.ninemile.org/fulltext.htm>

This site has four authoritative medical journals that include international coverage: (1) *Emerging Infectious Diseases*, (2) *Journal of Experimental Medicine*, (3) *Journal of General Physiology*, and (4) *Morbidity and Mortality Weekly Report*.

SUMMARY

The ability to retrieve information on diseases and conditions from around the world is immensely useful. The World Wide Web has opened up a channel to allow us to do this in a timely and efficient manner. Many organizations have been trying to find a central way to communicate and share information among countries, on a global basis, for a long time. The Web has allowed organizations such as WHO and the U.S. Agency for International Development finally to find a forum to do this. Still other organizations, such as Outbreak and SatelLife, have come into being because of the effective communication abilities that the World Wide Web has to offer. As health sciences librarians, the Web continuously offers us new ways to find information on diseases and conditions from other parts of the globe that were not made available to us before. Also, we have the opportunity to use the Web to share our information with other countries who are in need of it.

What is the status of the World Wide Web in other countries around the world? Is Web penetration worldwide significant enough to make medical information collaboration effective right now? A leading online consultant in Europe, Nua, has conducted surveys around the globe to discover the penetration of the Internet in other countries. In Brazil, the total online population was estimated to be at 1 million in 1997.[1] In Italy, Nua reports that 1.1 percent of Italian families (216,000) have home access to the Internet, and over 300 Internet Service Providers compete for their business.[2] In March 1997, Nua reported that Japan had 3.5 million users on the Web.[3] Another Nua report from July 1997 noted that 80,000 people in India currently use the Internet, and the number was expected to increase to 1.5 million by 2000.[4] Last, over 600,000 persons in

South Africa were found to have Internet access.[5] The Internet is slowly reaching out across the globe, although for the most part it is still distributed through North America, Western Europe, and Asia (Japan).[6]

As of August 1999, the number of Web users worldwide is estimated to be at 195 million, and is predicted to be 500 million by the year 2003 and 717 million by the year 2005.[7] In 1996, there were 5,511,000,000 personal computers in existence around the world. By the year 2000, this number is expected to grow to 16,200,000,000.[8]

Because of the presence of the World Wide Web and the continuously growing availability of communications technology around the world, we may look forward to a future where every nation and geographic location on the globe can enjoy unrestricted access to medical information when they need it.

REFERENCE NOTES

1. Nua Internet Surveys, November 4, 1997. Available: <http://www.nua.net/surveys>.

2. Nua Internet Surveys, February 11, 1998. Available: <http://www.nua.net/surveys>.

3. Nua Internet Surveys, October 31, 1997. Available: <http://www.nua.net/surveys>.

4. Nua Internet Surveys, July 14, 1997. Available: <http://www.nua.net/surveys>.

5., Nua Internet Surveys, October 20, 1997. Available: <http://www.nua.net/surveys>.

6. "High-level Access; Increase in Demand for Internet Connection." *Computer Industry Report*, 32(November 1, 1997) (16/17): 6.

7. Nua Internet Surveys, September 10, 1999. Available: <http://www.nua.net/surveys>.

8. International Data Corporation, 1997.

Index

Page numbers followed by the letter "t" indicate tables.

Eurosurveillance Weekly (Web site),
  156
Evaluating information, 28-30,
  83-85, 101, 104-106, 123-126
Evidence-based medicine, 67-73
  cause or harm, 70-72
  diagnosis, 68-70, 71t
  prognosis, 73, 74t
  therapy, 68, 69t
Excite, 14, 118-9, 120t
Excite Web Search, 94

Federal Web Locator (Web site), 135
FEDSTATS (Web site), 144
FEDWORLD (Web site), 135
Field searching
  body, 23-24
  citation searching, 24
  title, 23
  URL, 24
Finding Government Information:
  What's the Difference? (Web
  site), 147
Finding Government Information on
  the Internet: A Hands on
  Workshop (Web site), 147
Food and Drug Administration (Web
  site), 138
Friends of NLM, 7
Full-text journals. *See* Electronic
  journals
Fuzzy logic, 20

Galaxy, 15
Gateway sites, 80
Go Ask Alice! (Newsgroup), 106
Gopher, 16
GovBot (Web site), 135
Government resources, 129-148
  print resources, 131-133
  use of search engines, 133-134
  Web sources, 133-147
GPO Access (Web site), 145

GPO Browse Topics (Web site), 136
GPO Monthly Catalog (Web site),
  136
GPO Pathway Services (Web site),
  136
Grateful Med. *See* Internet Grateful
  Med
*Greenbook Overview of Entitlement
  Programs Committee on Ways
  and Means* (Web site), 151

Hardin Meta Directory of Internet
  Health (Web site), 19, 42-43,
  80, 89, 91-92
*Health, United States 1998 with
  Socioeconomic Status and
  Health Chartbook* (Web site),
  152
Health, United States Series (Web
  site), 152
Health Care Financing
  Administration (Web site),
  138, 161
Health Information Technology
  Institute of Mitretek Systems,
  Inc., 4
Health Oasis: Mayo Clinic. *See*
  Mayo Clinic Health Oasis
  (Web site)
Health on the Net (HON) Foundation,
  4, 28-29, 125-126. *See also*
  HON Code of Conduct; HON
  Principles
Health Resources and Services
  Administration (Web site),
  138-139
Health Statistics Page. Falk Library
  of the Health Sciences
  (University of Pittsburgh)
  (Web site), 162
HealthAtoZ (Web site), 37-38, 80, 107
Healthfinder (Web site), 6, 15, 37,
  80, 86-87, 90, 103, 121
  online journals, 173-174

HAWORTH Medical Information Sources
Sandra Wood, MLS, MBA
Senior Editor

HEALTH CARE RESOURCES ON THE INTERNET: A GUIDE FOR LIBRARI-ANS AND HEALTH CARE CONSUMERS edited by M. Sandra Wood. (2000). "A practical guide and an essential research tool to the Internet's vast and varied resources for health care has arrived —and its voice is professional and accessible. . . . This comprehensive work is an important reference tool that is readable and enjoyable." *Elizabeth (Betty) R. Warner, MSLS, AHIP, Coordinator of Information Literacy Programs, Academic Information Services and Research, Thomas Jefferson University, Philadelphia, Pennsylvania*

EATING POSITIVE: A NUTRITION GUIDE AND RECIPE BOOK FOR PEOPLE WITH HIV/AIDS by Jeffrey T. Huber and Kris Riddlesperger. (1998). "Four stars! . . . A much-needed book that could have a positive impact on the quality of life for persons with HIV/AIDS. . . . Many of the recipes are old favorites that have been enhanced for the person with HIV. . . . All people with nutritional problems may also find this book helpful. It is not reserved solely for the person with HIV/AIDS." *Doody Publishing, Inc.*

HIV/AIDS AND HIV/AIDS-RELATED TERMINOLOGY: A MEANS OF ORGA-NIZING THE BODY OF KNOWLEDGE by Jeffrey T. Huber and Mary L. Gillaspy. (1996). "Provides the needed standardized terminology to describe large HIV/AIDS collections. . . . A welcome book for any cataloger, indexer, or archivist who is faced with organizing a mass of information that is growing very rapidly. . . . highly recommended for all librarians with extensive collections." *Booklist: Reference Books Bulletin*

HIV/AIDS COMMUNITY INFORMATION SERVICES: EXPERIENCES IN SERVING BOTH AT-RISK AND HIV-INFECTED POPULATIONS by Jeffrey T. Huber. (1996). "Provides a well-organized introduction to HIV/AIDS information services that will be useful to those affected by HIV disease, health care practitioners, librarians, and other information professionals. Appropriate for all libraries and an excellent reference resource." *CHOICE*

USER EDUCATION IN HEALTH SCIENCES LIBRARIES: A READER edited by M. Sandra Wood. (1995). "A welcome addition to any health sciences library collection. A valuable tool for both academic and hospital librarians, as well as library school students interested in bibliographic instruction." *National Network*

CD-ROM IMPLEMENTATION AND NETWORKING IN HEALTH SCIENCES LIBRARIES edited by M. Sandra Wood. (1993). "Neatly compacts information about the history, selection, and management of CD-ROM technology in libraries. . . . Librarians at all levels of CD-ROM implementation can benefit from the solutions and ideas presented." *Bulletin of the Medical Library Association*

HOW TO FIND INFORMATION ABOUT AIDS, SECOND EDITION edited by Jeffrey T. Huber. (1992). "Since organizations and sources in this field are constantly changing, this updated edition is welcome. . . . A valuable resource for health or medical and public library collections." *Booklist: Reference Books Bulletin*

Order Your Own Copy of
This Important Book for Your Personal Library!

HEALTH CARE RESOURCES ON THE INTERNET
A Guide for Librarians and Health Care Consumers

_____ in hardbound at $39.95 (ISBN: 0-7890-0632-4)

_____ in softbound at $24.95 (ISBN: 0-7890-0911-0)

COST OF BOOKS_____

OUTSIDE USA/CANADA/
MEXICO: ADD 20%_____

POSTAGE & HANDLING_____
(US: $3.00 for first book & $1.25
for each additional book)
Outside US: $4.75 for first book
& $1.75 for each additional book)

SUBTOTAL_____

IN CANADA: ADD 7% GST_____

STATE TAX_____
(NY, OH & MN residents, please
add appropriate local sales tax)

FINAL TOTAL_____
(If paying in Canadian funds,
convert using the current
exchange rate. UNESCO
coupons welcome.)

☐ **BILL ME LATER:** ($5 service charge will be added)
(Bill-me option is good on US/Canada/Mexico orders only;
not good to jobbers, wholesalers, or subscription agencies.)

☐ Check here if billing address is different from
shipping address and attach purchase order and
billing address information.

Signature_____

☐ **PAYMENT ENCLOSED:** $_____

☐ **PLEASE CHARGE TO MY CREDIT CARD.**

☐ Visa   ☐ MasterCard   ☐ AmEx   ☐ Discover
☐ Diner's Club

Account # _____

Exp. Date _____

Signature _____

Prices in US dollars and subject to change without notice.

NAME _____

INSTITUTION _____

ADDRESS _____

CITY _____

STATE/ZIP _____

COUNTRY _____ COUNTY (NY residents only) _____

TEL _____ FAX _____

E-MAIL_____
May we use your e-mail address for confirmations and other types of information? ☐ Yes   ☐ No

Order From Your Local Bookstore or Directly From
The Haworth Press, Inc.
10 Alice Street, Binghamton, New York 13904-1580 • USA
TELEPHONE: 1-800-HAWORTH (1-800-429-6784) / Outside US/Canada: (607) 722-5857
FAX: 1-800-895-0582 / Outside US/Canada: (607) 772-6362
E-mail: getinfo@haworthpressinc.com
PLEASE PHOTOCOPY THIS FORM FOR YOUR PERSONAL USE.

BOF96